lymphedema

"At a time when few resources exist, this book responds to a
need voiced so desperately by women with breast cancer.
The book is incredibly well-written—concise and easy to
read—and able to get across exactly the information that
patients want. The practical knowledge and guidance through
management options satisfies all possible readers. An
emphatic and empowering tone are apparent throughout the
book.

"Besides being a welcome addition to any resource
library, this is a good recommendation for patients to add to
their personal library. The low cost makes this information
accessible to many people and a real find."
— *Oncology Nursing Forum*

"If you are one of thousands of women who suffer from
lymphedema, a common complication of breast cancer
surgery and treatment, take heart. Hunter House has just
released *Lymphedema*, the first book to provide clear information about this chronic condition, describe specific
treatment techniques, and-perhaps most important—show
women that relief lies within their own hands.

"The authors know whereof they speak: Jeannie Burt is a
breast cancer survivor and lymphedema patient; Gwen White
is her physical therapist. Their text is thorough and readable,
offering practical lessons in healing.

"While it sheds light on a generally overlooked condition,
this book's strength lies not only in its content, but in the
spirit of hope it engenders."
— *MAMM*

more reviewer comments on the next page...

"[The authors] have written a book focused on patient education and empowerment while compiling a wide range of information and expertise that offers an excellent resource to clinicians."

— Physical Therapy

"For me personally, ... the book validated the treatment I ... received for my cancer. In addition, I felt a renewed sense of appreciation for the care I received and for my good fortune to have been treated by caring physicians who were so thorough about all aspects and ramifications of my cancer."

— The Permanente Journal

Ordering

Trade bookstores in the U.S. and Canada please contact:

Publishers Group West
1700 Fourth Street, Berkeley CA 94710
Phone: (800) 788-3123   Fax: (800) 351-5073

Hunter House books are available at bulk discounts for textbook course adoptions; to qualifying community, health-care, and government organizations; and for special promotions and fund-raising. For details please contact:

Special Sales Department
Hunter House Inc., PO Box 2914, Alameda CA 94501-0914
Phone: (510) 865-5282   Fax: (510) 865-4295
E-mail: ordering@hunterhouse.com

Individuals can order our books from most bookstores, by calling (800) 266-5592, or from our website at www.hunterhouse.com

Lymphedema

a
BREAST CANCER PATIENT'S
GUIDE *to* PREVENTION
and HEALING

second edition

Jeannie Burt & Gwen White, P.T.

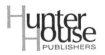

Hunter House PUBLISHERS

Hunter House Inc., Publishers
PO Box 2914
Alameda CA 94501-0914

Library of Congress Cataloging-in-Publication Data

Burt, Jeannie.
Lymphedema : a breast cancer patient's guide to prevention and healing / Jeannie Burt and Gwen White.— 2nd ed.
p. cm.
Summary: "Describes options women have for preventing and treating lymphedema, a swelling condition that may occur after breast cancer surgery"—Provided by publisher.
Includes bibliographical references and index.
ISBN-13: 978-0-89793-458-9 (pbk.)
ISBN-10: 0-89793-458-X (pbk.)
1. Lymphedema. 2. Breast—Cancer—Treatment—Complications. I. White, Gwen, P.T. II. Title.
RC646.3.B87 2005
616.99'446059—dc22   2005013581

Project Credits

Cover Design: Kathy Warinner
Illustrations: Kathy Albert
Book Design & Production: Hunter House
Developmental and Copy Editor: Kelley Blewster
Indexer: Nancy D. Peterson
Acquisitions Editor: Jeanne Brondino
Editor: Alexandra Mummery
Publishing Assistants: Antonia T. Lee & Herman Leung
Publishing Intern: Shelley McGuire
Publicist: Jillian Steinberger
Customer Service Manager: Christina Sverdrup
Order Fulfillment: Joe Winebarger, Washul Lakdhon
Administrator: Theresa Nelson
Computer Support: Peter Eichelberger
Publisher: Kiran S. Rana

Manufactured in the United States of America

7 6 5 4 3   Second Edition   10 11 12 13

contents

part two   Treating Lymphedema

─────────────── **Important Note** ───────────────

The material in this book is intended to provide a review of information regarding lymphedema and its treatment. Every effort has been made to provide accurate and dependable information. The contents of this book have been compiled through professional research and in consultation with medical professionals. However, health-care professionals have differing opinions, and advances in medical and scientific research are made very quickly, so some of the information may become outdated.

Therefore, the publisher, authors, and editors, as well as any professionals quoted in the book, cannot be held responsible for any error, omission, or dated material. The authors and publisher assume no responsibility for any outcome of applying the information in this book in a program of self-care or under the care of a licensed practitioner. If you have questions about the application of the information described in this book, consult a qualified health-care professional.

foreword

I am delighted to be asked to write a foreword to this book.

Lymphedema has long been a largely ignored complication following cancer. Some people are simply born with lymphatic insufficiency and may have had the condition for many years. In most cases, patients have been told that lymphedema is something they just have to live with and that nothing can be done for them. This is simply not true.

As our knowledge has grown over the years, treatment procedures have greatly improved, and so has our understanding of the disease. Diagnostic techniques have been greatly developed, and there is an increased awareness of the condition on the part of both the medical profession and the public in general.

Early diagnosis and an immediate treatment course with carefully individualized education on self-management are essential. Maintaining this self-care will lead to further reduction, and will take only a short time on a daily basis. This means that the focus of the patient's life will not be on her lymphedema, but on what she can achieve and enjoy without further complications. With compliance and self-care, a positive outcome, in terms of both self-esteem and well-being, lies in the patient's own hands.

Patient support groups now exist worldwide. The Lymphoedema Association of Australia (L.A.A.) was one of the first to be formed (in 1982), and our first large patient meeting was held in Adelaide, Australia, at the International Society of Lymphology congress in 1985. Knowledge regarding patient care and treatment has spread to most countries of the world, and Internet sites provide valuable resources. This book is an important publication from a number of points of view.

First, it gives clear information on what lymphedema is and why it occurs. Second, it describes treatment procedures to suit a range of needs, and it emphasizes that lymphedema can be treated successfully. Of even more value, it gives patients hope for their future. They will know after reading this book that they are not alone and that there are many avenues of help and support available.

I congratulate the authors for their persistence in this project and on a work well done. I wish it every success. I am sure it will be extremely useful to people with lymphedema and will give them hope and courage to manage their condition better. This condition must not rule patients' lives; with care and understanding of their condition, people with lymphedema can live a full life.

— *Judith R. Casley-Smith, M.D.*
Malvern, Australia

acknowledgments

Bringing a book like this to fruition would not be possible without the efforts and guidance of many people, and we wish to thank everyone who helped make this book a reality. We are especially grateful for the support, encouragement, and expertise of Drs. Stephen Chandler, James Schwarz, Daniel Ladizinsky, Wayne Gilbert, Jai Nautiyal, Edythe Vickers, Judith R. Casley Smith, and Robert Lerner. We owe a debt of gratitude to the professionalism and vision of Saskia R. J. Thiadens, R.N.; Ruth Bach, M.Ed., L.P.C.; Izetta Smith, M.A.; Vicki Romm, L.C.S.W.; Fern Carness, MPH, R.N.; Ruth Coopee, MOT, OTR/CHT, MLD/CKT; and Kristie Lackey, PTA.

We also want to thank Joan Weddle, Shirley Schreiner, Kathryn Tierney, Nancy Espinoza, R.N., Barbara Henarie, Julene Fox, Nancy Friedemann, R.N.,Vera Wheeler, R.N., and Emma Garza for the gifts of their time and experience. Without their generosity this book would not have been possible.

We must thank the following people for the knowledge they've imparted about lymphedema: the Vodders, who developed the first treatments; the Foeldis, who made treatment techniques more widely available; Drs. John R. and Judith Casley-Smith, whose Lymphoedema Association of Australia conducts worldwide research and education; Dr. Robert Lerner, a pioneer in bringing lymphedema treatment and training programs to the United States; Drs. Charles and Marlys Witte, for their support of research with the International Society of Lymphology; and Saskia Thiadens, who has dedicated years to championing lymphedema education and has provided a means through which practitioners can communicate with each other by founding the National Lymphedema Network.

preface

We wrote this book with the goal that it be clear and helpful to patients and their families. We wanted it to be easily understood, since we realized that most people reading it wouldn't have a medical vocabulary. Unavoidably, however, some of the material is pretty technical, especially in the first three chapters, which contain a lot of information about physiology. Still, dear reader, please realize that you don't need to understand every bit of information presented here to be able to learn and apply techniques that can prevent or treat lymphedema or give you ways to live with it. If you wish, skim some of the heavier material. Even without a thorough understanding of it all, you can learn what counts for your health.

We worked as a team, but each of us focused on the parts of the book that better fit our specialites. Gwen White, who has over thirty years' experience as a physical therapist, wrote the technical chapters; Jeannie Burt, who has lymphedema, wrote the case studies and some of the later chapters. Below are our individual stories as they led to the book, as well as information about our consultants on the project.

We hope you will find this book both informative and comforting. We also hope it will give you a means to find help for your lymphedema so you can deal with it and release whatever hold it has on your life. Read on. There is help, and with help there is hope.

Jeannie Burt's Story

I know about lymphedema. I have had it since May of 1997, just weeks after I finished chemotherapy and radiation for breast cancer.

The swelling was gradual at first, and I thought it would go away. Then, one hot, humid weekend, after I'd transplanted a patch of overgrown daisies, it just ballooned. My whole arm looked like it was smothered in lumpy white flesh. My shoulder began to ache. My elbow became bloated and fiery hot.

On Monday I tried to call my oncologist. The receptionist said he was gone for a week. A week! A lifetime! I tried to tell myself I could wait for the doctor to return, that everything would be okay. But in truth I started to panic. At night I couldn't sleep. My imagination kicked in like it hadn't since I was a child conjuring demons. How much more lopsided and huge would I get before I could talk to my doctor? I'd hold up my arm and shake it. I felt totally out of control. The bed sheets would knot around me as I squeezed my elbow and did some exercises with my hand. But in the morning my arm would still be swollen.

I was turning into a witch consumed with worry. My parents called from their farm three hundred miles away. I told them about the swelling, then flew into a tirade when they didn't give it the concern I thought it deserved. My husband was worried and puzzled and looked as though he too felt helpless. He held my hand and just let me rant. No one seemed to understand why, after all I'd gone through with cancer, this was bothering me so much. But it was.

I couldn't wait for my doctor's return. I had to do something, to take some kind of action. I decided to find out as much as possible about what could be causing the swelling, so I dug around in the large stack of papers the clinic had given me when I'd first been diagnosed with breast cancer. I looked through pages on chemo drugs, a booklet on arranging hats and scarves on a head with no hair, reams of disclaimers, instructions on what not to eat before surgery. Yet there was just one measly line mentioning possible swelling, and it gave the swelling a name: lymphedema. When my husband came home that day after work, I waved the sheet of paper in his face and screamed, "At least I have a name for it!" I went to the library. I'd be exaggerating if I said the library had next to nothing on lymphedema. Two books on breast cancer mentioned it, for a total of three paragraphs. Both books said there wasn't much to do about it.

I felt totally lost and hopeless. Self-pity is not normally a big emotion for me. Well, let me tell you, I was wallowing in it.

My oncologist finally got back from his trip. His voice over the phone sounded kind and calm. He told me about Gwen, a physcial therapist who specialized in lymphedema, and assured me there were new techniques for dealing with it. I have since realized how lucky I was that my doctor knew about lymphedema and knew how to get help for me. Most doctors, it seems, still don't know about the help that is available.

My course of therapy began. Gwen not only treated my lymphedema but also instructed me in helping myself. Knowing what to do gave me back my sense of power and control. And Gwen didn't stop with helping only me, but willingly took time from her tremendously busy life to cowrite this book so that others might not have to feel at such an awful loss as I once did.

My life now is where I want it to be. Though my arm has not completely returned to the size and shape it used to be, I think I have the tools to make it so if I want to put the time and effort into it. Lymphedema is no longer a demanding voice in my life, merely a whisper. I don't think a stranger would know I ever had lymphedema. I know I will always be vulnerable to another episode of swelling, so I'm still careful to follow Gwen's instructions. It's not a bad outcome.

If you have lymphedema or are just concerned about its potential, please read on. If someone—your doctor, your nurse, anyone—tells you there is nothing to do about the condition, don't believe them. There's plenty you can do, my friend. The information in this book should help you.

Gwen White's Story

I recall the first time I ever heard the term *manual lymph drainage*. It was in 1996 and I had been a physical therapist for over twenty-two years. I worked in a temporomandibular-joint disorders (TMJ) clinic with patients who suffered head and facial pain. I was also a health educator. My third (and most important) job was being a mother to three children, who at the time were all under eleven years old. One day at a staff meeting, my boss said the oncology department in our

HMO was pressuring him to train a therapist to provide a new treat-ment—lymphatic massage—for patients with lymphedema. Evi-dently some well-informed patients had been insisting on receiving the therapy. My boss asked for a volunteer. My cup felt pretty full (in fact, at times it seemed to runneth over), and volunteering crossed my mind for only a second as I wondered what this treatment was and who would want to work with people who'd had cancer.

No one volunteered. My boss said someone on our staff *would* be going down to Anaheim the following week for an all-expenses-paid, four-day training in lymphedema management for breast can-cer patients, and he would pick someone if there were no volunteers. I mentally reviewed my schedule, my kids' schedules, and my hus-band's schedule and decided that I could potentially arrange to go. My hand went up. I thought I could really use a break from my regu-lar schedule, and four days at the Hyatt Regency sounded wonder-ful, whatever this lymphatic massage stuff was.

The twist of fate that resulted from my raising my hand that day has taken me on a fascinating journey. It is funny how some-times when a door opens, if we take a reluctant step through it, we find something unexpected and wonderful. Working with lym-phedema has been one of the more exciting things I have done. I have been challenged and stimulated as never before. I completed the Vodder certification through the Dr. Vodder School of North America, have attended recertification classes several times, and have passed the Lymphedema Association of North American (LANA) certification for lymphedema therapists. I have attended breast cancer conferences, several National Lymphedema Network conferences, many different lymphedema workshops, and courses on myofascial release, scar work, Kinesiotaping, bandaging, and pa-tient support. I joined a local group of lymphedema therapists who meet monthly. I have been reading everything I can about lym-phedema (the amount of which is growing every year), have given many talks and in-service trainings about lymphedema to a variety of groups (both professionals and patients), and have developed two lymphedema programs—one in the large HMO that trained and supported me as I learned about the condition, and a second in the small physical therapy clinic my husband owns. I cowrote this book, and now am updating it with all the things I have learned in the past six years. Hopefully this second edition will offer even greater benefit to its readers.

I have been privileged to work for the past several years with a wonderful physical therapist assistant, Kristie Lackey, who also became LANA certified. I have learned a lot from her insights and her creative problem solving. My work as a lymphedema therapist continues to thrill me. I have never worked with tools and techniques so effective (they work for almost everyone) and so necessary for a group of patients who previously had few ways to help themselves. It is exciting to work with patients who are motivated in their treatment. I came to realize that patients who have had cancer are very special people. Many have truly been transformed by their experiences and view the world differently. It has been a gift to meet and work with so many of them.

I have received gratifying feedback from therapists all over the world who recommend this book to their patients and who tell me how helpful it has been. It warms my heart when patients tell me how much they appreciate the book or how it helped them to better understand lymphedema and reassured them that they could do something about it. That was the reason why Jeannie and I wrote the book in the first place: so people could easily access some simple tools that could help them right away.

As you read *Lymphedema*, our hope is that you will find something that can help you. Find the parts of the book that apply to you, try different things, and see what works. Perhaps you will see yourself in some of the stories; perhaps you just want to learn aspects of self-care; perhaps you will read every bit of the medical information as well. Lymphedema treatment is not an exact science, and what helps one person may not help the next. No two patients, or their needs and goals, are exactly the same. Our belief is that each person should learn as much as possible to better understand the illness and the treatments that are available. Then do what is necessary to effectively manage your condition at a level that is right for you, so you can get on with your life. Make your management of lymphedema fit you and your situation.

About the Consultants for This Book

Stephen Chandler, M.D., attended the McGill University Medical School in Montreal and completed an internship while on rotation at the University of California County Hospitals. He spent three years during the Vietnam War as a flight surgeon on air evacuations. He completed a residency in internal medicine at the Oregon Health and Science University (OHSU), where he also had a fellowship in hematology. In addition to practicing as an oncologist, he administers to peoples of other countries through groups such as Physicians for Social Responsibility and Northwest Medical Teams. In this role he has traveled to Jamaica, Bolivia, Nicaragua, Russia, Botswana, and Finland.

James A. Schwarz, M.D., attended college at Princeton University, received his medical degree from the University of California in San Francisco, and completed his surgical residency at Stanford University. He continued with a fellowship in surgery oncology at Roswell Park Cancer Institute, in Buffalo, New York. Since 1988, he has had a general surgery practice in San Jose, California, and in Oregon. The largest portion of his practice serves oncology patients.

Edythe Vickers, N.D., L.Ac., B.Sc., earned her bachelor's degree from the University of Toronto, her license in the field of acupuncture and Chinese herbs from the Oregon College of Oriental Medicine in 1986, and her degree in naturopathic medicine at the National College of Naturopathic Medicine in 1987. She has been practicing since 1987.

Wayne Gilbert, M.D., attended medical school at St. Louis University, completed his internship at Oregon Health and Science University, and did his surgical residency at Legacy Emanuel Hospital and Health Center and the Kaiser Residency Program in Portland, Oregon. He has been practicing general surgery for ten years.

Jai Nautiyal, M.D., attended the University of Chicago Medical School. He completed his residency at the University of Chicago, where he later practiced for seven years in the Department of Radiation and Cellular Oncology. He currently practices with Radiation Oncologists, P.C., in Portland, Oregon.

Daniel Ladizinsky, M.D., attended the University of Michigan Medical School. He completed a surgical residency at the University of Arizona College of Medicine, where he trained with Drs. Charles and Marlys Witte, who founded the Intenational Society of Lymphology. He currently practices plastic surgery in Oregon.

part one

LYMPHEDEMA: WHAT IT IS *and* HOW *to* PREVENT IT

1

the BASICS about
LYMPHEDEMA

The human lymphatic system is vast and extremely complex. In this chapter we discuss the basics about the lymphatic system and about lymphedema in terms that can be understood by almost everyone. Even with the focus on simplicity, however, the discussion is somewhat technical. Do not be discouraged if it doesn't make complete sense. In later chapters, you will see that understanding the lymphatic system in detail is not essential to successfully dealing with lymphedema. Skim these first few chapters if you like, and read them again later when you can take everything in.

What Is Lymphedema?

Lymphedema is swelling, usually in the arms or legs, that occurs as a result of an impaired lymphatic system (see Figure 1.1). A person's lymphatic system can be impaired in a variety of ways: by surgery, radiotherapy, injury, or even infection. The impairment can also occur simply as a result of the makeup of the person's genes.

The lymphatic system is part of both the immune system and the circulatory system. You will see in more detail in a later chapter that it is responsible for cleansing the body's tissues and maintaining its balance of fluids. Specifically, the vessels that make up the lymphatic system drain excess fluid from the body's cells, along with protein molecules, bacteria, viruses, cellular waste products, and other unusable matter. Once this protein-rich fluid called *lymph* has entered the lymphatic system, it is transported through the lymphatic vessels to the lymph nodes, where it is filtered and cleansed of the waste products and other materials it carried out of the cells. Eventually the lymph fluid rejoins the blood by flowing into the large veins just before they enter the heart. Unlike the blood circulatory system, which carries blood both toward the heart and away from it, the lymphatic system is a "one-way" system; that is, it carries its fluid away from the body's cells *toward* the heart.

If the lymphatic system has been impaired, the lymph fluid can back up. Swelling, or lymphedema, occurs when the amount of fluid in an area is greater than the capacity of the lymphatic system to transport it away. Lymphedema has also been defined as "an abnormal accumulation of tissue proteins, edema, and chronic inflammation within an extremity."[1] If the condition is left untreated, the

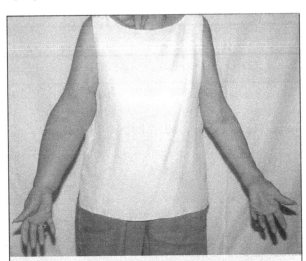

Figure 1.1. *Patient with lymphedema of the right arm*

excess of protein-rich lymph fluid can provide a breeding ground for bacteria that can result in infection and can delay wound healing, because less oxygen gets to the tissue cells.[2] A long-term accumulation of lymph fluid eventually causes tissues to thicken and harden (a condition called *fibrosis*), which creates further resistance to the draining of fluid from the limb.

If a person's lymph nodes are removed or radiated as a part of cancer treatment, she or he will be at risk of developing lymphedema for the rest of her or his life. Some breast cancer survivors—about half—will never get visible lymphedema at all. In others, the swelling starts immediately following surgery or radiotherapy. For others, it may not appear until many years later.[3] Still others may endure an episode of lymphedema that lasts for a few weeks, disappears, and may or may not ever return.

Causes and Types of Lymphedema

Lymphedema can occur in anyone—man, woman, or child—from any of several different causes. It can occur anywhere in the body but is most common in the arms, legs, and breast tissue.

Some of the causes of lymphedema are[4]

* surgery, particularly when lymph nodes are removed during treatment for cancer of the following types: breast, prostate, gynecological, head or neck, colon, melanoma, or sarcoma

* radiotherapy, which kills tumor cells but can also produce scar tissue, which in turn can interrupt the normal flow of the lymphatic system

* trauma that disrupts an area of the body containing lymph nodes

* infection, including lymphangitis (inflammation or infection of the lymph vessels themselves)

* cancer, which itself can block lymph flow

* filariasis, a disease found mostly in endemic areas of Southeast Asia, India, and Africa, and caused by parasitic worms called *filaria* that enter the lymphatic vessels that lie close to the body's surface

* paralysis or immobility

* chronic venous insufficiency (abnormally low return of blood from the legs to the trunk by way of the veins)

* obesity

When lymphedema results from any of these causes it is known as *secondary lymphedema*. In each case, the chance of developing the condition can be increased by certain contributing factors. These can range from an extensive trauma to a small, inconsequential injury, such as the kind that results from a cat scratch, a bug bite, or everyday activities like gardening or household chores. Even a hot day or an airplane flight can sometimes trigger an episode. A lymphedema patient who came into Gwen's clinic had undergone bilateral mastectomies—the first in 1957, the second in 1964. She had experienced no swelling problems for thirty-three years; in fact, she had no idea she even had a chance of developing lymphedema. Then, during a hot summer day when she was packing and lifting boxes to prepare for a move, her arm suddenly started to swell. Although we'll never be sure, this woman might have been able to avoid developing lymphedema if she had spaced her heavy chores out over several days or done them during the coolest part of the day. Unfortunately, she had no way of knowing this. One of the goals of this book is to inform you about potential triggers of lymphedema and how to avoid them.

As mentioned above, not everyone who undergoes radiotherapy or the surgical removal of lymph nodes develops lymphedema. In many people the remaining lymphatics (lymph vessels) dilate or form collateral circulation or new pathways. Dr. James Schwarz, a surgeon Gwen works with, explains that the lymphatic system differs greatly from person to person. "This may help to explain why, of the many women who have the same surgery and treatment, some develop trouble with lymphedema and some don't," he says.

Another type of lymphedema—one not associated with surgery or radiotherapy—is caused by a malformation or malfunction of the lymphatic system, a condition known as *primary lymphedema*. It can be present at birth (Milroy's disease), develop at or around puberty (lymphedema praecox), or develop after age thirty-five (lymphedema tarda). It is most commonly related to having too few lymphatic vessels; it is unclear if people are born with this insufficiency or if it develops over time. Some suggest that the defect may be programmed at birth to cause atrophy or early aging in the lymphatic vessels, resulting in inadequate drainage.[3] In Milroy's disease, which is an inherited disorder, there is a complete absence of the initial lymph vessels (the microscopic vessels where fluid first enters the lymphatic system).[5] Primary lymphedema affects females more than males. In 95 percent of cases, swelling occurs in the legs, but it can develop anywhere in the body where structural abnormalities compromise lymph drainage. Primary lymphedema may be linked to heredity or to genetic syndromes, but it can also develop without any genetic component.

Almost all the treatment and recommendations suggested in this book can be applied to both primary and secondary lymphedema. However, we will be concentrating on secondary lymphedema, particularly when it is found in the upper body and occurs after treatment for breast cancer.

Breast Cancer Surgery and the Lymph Nodes

From the early 1900s until recent decades, the standard treatment for breast cancer was a *radical mastectomy*: removal of the breast, the muscles of the chest wall, and sometimes the underlying tissues, the surrounding skin, and the lymph nodes located in the armpit and above the collarbone. This extensive procedure decreased the local recurrence of cancer and increased survival rates. In recent decades, treatment has evolved toward more conservative surgery. Two surgeries that are currently common are modified radical mastectomy and breast-conserving (or breast-conservation) surgery. *Modified radical mastectomy* involves removal of only the breast and the axillary (armpit-area) lymph nodes. *Breast-conserving surgery*, also called *lumpectomy*, involves removal of only the localized tumor and the axillary lymph nodes; it is usually followed by radiotherapy and/or chemotherapy. In either case, the removal of the armpit-area lymph nodes is termed *axillary node dissection*. More recently, doctors have been combining lumpectomy with a procedure known as *sentinel lymph node biopsy*, followed by chemotherapy and/or radiotherapy.[6]

Let's take a closer look at some of the procedures described above.

Mastectomy

As mentioned, modified radical mastectomy involves removing the entire breast as well as the lymph nodes in the armpit. Doctors at the facility where Gwen works estimate that 20 to 30 percent of breast cancer surgeries currently being performed are modified radical mastectomies. If the removed lymph nodes do not show any evidence of cancer, radiation is unnecessary. But some cancer patients have nodes that contain cancer cells. Dr. Schwarz explains that if four or more lymph nodes test positive for cancer, radiation is recommended. Studies are underway to determine the best protocol to follow when fewer than four lymph nodes test positive for cancer.

Several factors can make a mastectomy preferable to a breast-conservation surgery. Some of them are

* multiple tumors in the same breast

* a large tumor, especially in a small breast

* a patient who does not want or cannot tolerate radiation

* cancer of the type termed *inflammatory breast cancer*

* the desire of the patient

Dr. Schwarz says one reason why a patient may request a mastectomy rather than a lumpectomy is if she has a medical history that puts her at higher risk for cancer—for example, someone who had Hodgkin's disease as a child and who wants to reduce her risk of breast cancer in the future. But reasons for choosing a mastectomy can vary widely. Gwen knows of a breast cancer patient who requested a mastectomy because she was an avid hunter, and every time she fired her rifle it recoiled and bruised her breast.

Some women even request a mastectomy of the uninvolved side (the breast without cancer). Patients at high risk for recurrence of cancer, such as women who have the gene that predisposes them to cancer, may want to have the second breast removed to reduce the risk. When a mastectomy is performed on a breast considered cancer free, it is referred to as a *prophylactic* (preventive) mastectomy;

the procedure involved is usually a *simple mastectomy*. Lymph nodes are not normally removed in a simple mastectomy. Dr. Schwarz recommends that patients who want a prophylactic mastectomy wait until they have completed cancer treatment. He says removing a second, unaffected breast during surgery may cause prolonged healing time, which can delay adjuvant treatment. Adjuvant treatment—chemotherapy, radiation, or hormone therapy prescribed after surgery to ensure that breast cancer does not return—is best begun as soon as possible after surgery.

Axillary Node Dissection

Axillary node dissection, or removal of some of the lymph nodes in the area of the armpit, is performed in most types of breast cancer

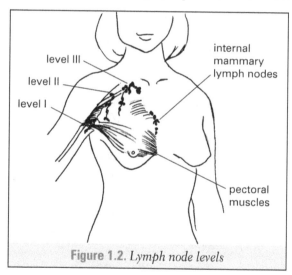

Figure 1.2. *Lymph node levels*

surgery to determine the progression of the cancer. Determining the extent and the charactistics of the cancer, a process called staging, helps the medical team decide which, if any, post-surgical treatments to recommend. The status of the axillary lymph nodes remains the single most important predictor of survival from breast cancer.[7]

Axillary lymph nodes are categorized as level I, II, or III, which roughly corresponds to their location in the underarm area (see Figure 1.2). Axillary node dissection can involve the nodes at any of these sites. In general, level I and sometimes level II nodes are removed during the procedure. Level III nodes are rarely removed. Dr. Schwarz explains why: "Removal of nodes at level III increases the risk of further destruction of lymphatics and [therefore] increases the risk of lymphedema. It is rarely done except in cases where levels I and II are highly involved in the cancer."

Axillary lymph node dissection can contribute to the development of lymphedema. It is commonly accepted that the greater the extent of lymph node dissection, the greater the risk of lymphedema.[8] Some women with lymphedema bemoan the fact that doctors removed their lymph nodes only to find an absence of cancer in the nodes. Still, evidence shows that even when lymph nodes test negative for cancer, axillary node dissection can increase survival rates.[9]

Some situations require no removal of lymph nodes at all, such as when the cancer is a small carcinoma in situ (cancer that has not spread to neighboring tissues). In this case, the risk of lymph node involvement is less than 1 percent. Dr. Schwarz says there are other cases in which axillary node dissection may not be recommended, for example, if the patient is an elderly woman with a slow-growing tumor.

Sentinel Node Biopsy

In recent years, sentinel node biopsy (SNB or SLNB), which provides an alternative to a complete axillary node dissection, has been a major advance in the treatment of breast cancer. In this procedure, either a blue dye or a sulfur colloid is injected into the breast around the site of the original tumor. The dye travels through the lymph vessels to the first (and often the second) lymph node in the axillary bed of nodes. The first lymph node, the sentinel node—plus often an additional node or two—is then surgically removed and examined for cancer by a pathologist while the patient is still in surgery. The idea behind the procedure is that the lymph nodes most susceptible to a spread of cancer would be the first ones that the lymphatic vessels travel to from the site of the tumor. If there is no evidence of cancer in the sentinel node(s), no more nodes are removed and axillary node dissection can be avoided.

A number of studies have confirmed that the absence of metastasis (the spread of cancer) in the sentinel node reliably predicts the absence of metastasis in the remaining axillary nodes.[10] In particular,

SLNB can be a safe and accurate method of screening the axillary nodes for metastasis in women with a small breast cancer.[11] If the sentinal node does show evidence of cancer cells, a complete axillary node dissection can then be performed while the patient is still under anesthetic. In such a case, removing all the remaining lymph nodes is currently standard practice; however, it is not clear that doing so improves survival rates. Studies are currently underway to evaluate this issue.

Women who undergo SLNB experience significantly fewer problems after surgery than those who undergo axillary node dissection. Patients with SLNB experience less lymphedema, improved range of motion in their arms, less pain and numbness, and fewer seromas (pockets of swelling at the surgical site) than those with axillary node dissection.[10,12,13,14,15] Studies show that these benefits can continue for up to twelve months.[16,17] Patients who've undergone SLNB also experience fewer problems with axillary web syndrome (cording and tightening of tissue in the armpit) than patients who've had axillary node dissection.[18]

Surgeon Wayne Gilbert has been involved in sentinel lymph node research. At the health-maintenance organization where he works, SLNB combined with breast-conservation surgery has become standard practice for breast cancer patients who meet the criteria for that procedure.Of his patients who qualify for SLNB, he says about 80 percent choose SLNB over axillary node dissection. Some patients who qualify for SLNB, however, still choose to have the lymph nodes removed.

Doctors will not recommend SLNB in the following cases:

* When the breast cancer has been biopsied, in which case there may be existing scar tissue that makes it less amenable to accurate sentinel node biopsy

* When there is a large tumor or there are multiple sites of cancer

* When there is clinical evidence, based on a doctor's physical examination of the area, of axillary node involvement

＊ When the patient has undergone neoadjuvant chemotherapy (chemo given prior to surgery to shrink the tumor)

＊ During pregnancy or lactation

In general, the less treatment a breast cancer patient receives,
the less likely she is to get lymphedema. (See below for some statistics on the incidence of lymphedema following breast cancer treatment.) Fortunately, the trend of the past five years has been for
surgeons to perform fewer axillary lymph node dissections.[19] Yet, as
promising as SLNB is, it is not a perfect prediction of metastatic
cancer. Dr. Schwarz points out that tests conducted after sentinel
node biopsy are occasionally misleading. Sometimes a test con-
cludes that the sentinel node is cancer free, even though further
tests show cancer in other axillary lymph nodes (a scenario termed a
false negative). Studies have shown that when five or more nodes are
shown to have cancer, the rate of false-negative readings increases.[20]

Additionally, Dr. Schwarz says the success of any SLNB procedure depends partly on the experience of the surgeon and partly on
the characteristics of the primary tumor. Using SLNB is still somewhat of an art. He notes that situations have occurred where either
the surgeon failed to find the sentinel node or the lymphatics were
obstructed with metastatic disease, causing tracer material to mi-
grate or to bypass the sentinel node altogether.

Hopefully, continued improvements in SLNB will benefit the
process of diagnosis and decrease the incidence of lymphedema in
breast cancer survivors. SLNB is exciting progress in the field of
breast cancer surgery. Additional randomized trials are currently underway to further define its best use.

Radiotherapy

Radiotherapy, or treatment with radiation, is an essential therapy for
most patients who develop invasive breast cancer. It is well accepted
that radiation improves survival after breast cancer.[21] It doesn't prevent cancer, but it treats whatever residual cancer may remain in the
chest wall and lymph nodes after surgery and chemotherapy.

Who Is a Candidate for Radiation Treatment?

Radiotherapy protocols vary with each patient. Doctors weigh several factors when deciding whether to recommend the treatment. It is usually recommended for patients at high risk for recurrence of cancer, such as those who have large or aggressive tumors, those whose lymph nodes have cancer cells in them, and those who show microscopic residual disease left over after surgery. In most cases, when a lumpectomy is performed, radiotherapy is given to the rest of the breast tissue. Sometimes the axilla (armpit) will be treated as well. Most patients who receive radiation will experience some breast swelling, much of which will normally reduce as the patient heals from the effects of radiation. Some patients, however, will be left with residual lymphedema in the breast or on the side of the trunk under the arm.

Radiation and Lymphedema

Although radiotherapy reduces the risk that cancer will recur, it also increases the chance of developing lymphedema.[21] Dr. Jai Nautiyal, a radiation oncologist, says, "Radiation can lead to scarring and increased lymphostasis [pooling of lymph fluid]. The use of radiation after axillary dissection can further aggravate the scarring that occurs after the surgery and thereby increase the likelihood of lymphedema." In general, the more radiation that is given, the higher the incidence of lymphedema. Likewise, the more conservative the radiation treatment, the lower the incidence of lymphedema. (See the section on the incidence of lymphedema, below, for some statistics on lymphedema after radiation treatment.)

Dr. Nautiyal says that in the past five years, radiotherapy has been refined to more accurately pinpoint the most effective dosages of radiation and the areas to be irradiated. Doctors can limit the radiation to specific fields (areas), depending on the type, location, and extent of the cancer. New radiotherapy techniques are continually being evaluated. Preliminary research suggests that providing a higher radiation dose per session while reducing the length of treatment to three weeks may be as effective as a longer course of treatment. Investigators are also looking into partial breast irradiation.[22]

How Radiotherapy Affects the Lymphatic System

Lymph nodes are sensitive to the effects of radiation. Radiotherapy depletes the lymphocytes in the nodes and decreases the nodes' filtering and immune functions. (Lymphocytes are a type of white blood cell that are heavily involved in the proper functioning of the immune system.) The effects of radiation are long-term; the scarring process can continue for a year or more after treatment and, as a final insult to a system that is already compromied, can cause lymphedema to develop. On the brighter side, however, radiotherapy affects only the area where the lymph nodes have been treated, not the entire lymphatic system.

It is interesting to note that the lymphatic *vessels* are resistant to radiotherapy. Their structure and function remain intact even when irradiated.[21] However, a problem can arise if the surrounding tissue develops fibrosis (hardening), which interrupts the drainage of lymph vessels and can lead to lymphedema.

Radiation or Not? Weighing the Risks

Given the risk of lymphedema, people with breast cancer may question whether it is advisable to pursue radiation treatment. But, while cancer can kill, lymphedema very rarely does. With proper attention some lymphedema can be prevented, and what can't be prevented can be effectively managed with appropriate treatment. It cannot be emphasized too strongly that **the benefits of radiotherapy far outweigh the potential risks of lymphedema.** Research clearly shows that radiotherapy improves survival rates and enhances the benefits of chemotherapy after breast cancer surgery.[21]

Reconstruction after Mastectomy

For many breast cancer survivors, reconstruction after a mastectomy is an important step in the process of returning to a comfortable life. In this section we give a brief overview of a woman's choices regarding reconstruction and the effects the procedure can have on lymphedema.

Options for Reconstruction Procedures

Dr. Daniel Ladizinsky, a plastic surgeon with many years of experience performing reconstructive surgery, describes the options available for breast reconstruction:

* Saline implant, which sometimes requires placement of a tissue expander prior to the implant surgery

* Reconstruction with the body's own tissue, most commonly using either the trans rectus abdominus muscle, from the abdominal area (a procedure knonwn as a *TRAM flap*), or the latissimus dorsi muscle, from the back beneath the shoulder blade

* Reconstruction using both implant and body tissue if there is not enough tissue to create an acceptable match to the other breast

In addition to the primary surgery to reconstruct the breast itself, procedures are required to create a nipple and to have a tattoo applied to match the color of the natural nipple and areola (the area of darker skin surrounding the nipple). Some women will also require surgery on the other breast to create a better match between the size and shape of the two breasts. Surgery on the second breast may include a breast lift, a reduction, or a repositioning of the nipple.[23] The plastic surgeon will work with you to determine what procedures will give you the best outcome based on your anatomy and lifestyle.

Reconstruction and Radiation

If a patient *will not be* receiving radiation, reconstructive surgery can be performed immediately after breast cancer surgery. If a patient *will be* receiving radiotherapy, most authorities recommend delaying reconstruction until after the radiation treatment is completed. Undergoing reconstructive surgery before radiotherapy is not recommended because radiation may cause changes in the reconstructed breast significant enough to require more surgery. It can increase the risk of scarring, puckering, fibrosis (hardening), fat necrosis (a lump of hardened fatty-tissue cells), and flap contracture (shrinking and pulling of the body tissue used to create the breast).[24] Delaying breast reconstruction until after the patient has fully healed from radiotherapy will help to prevent some of these problems.[25]

Dr Ladizinsky reports that prior to 1998, approximately 80 percent of his surgeries for breast reconstruction were done immediately after the mastectomy. But research began to show a significant increase in survival rates for breast cancer patients when adjuvant radiotherapy was added to the treatment protocol.[26,27] Now only 10–15 percent of Dr. Ladizinsky's breast reconstruction surgeries are done immediately after mastectomy. As mentioned earlier, some mastectomy patients do not require radiation. The need for radiation depends on the type of cancer, the size and location of the tumor, and involvement of the axillary lymph nodes. However, these factors are usually not known until after the mastectomy and the staging of the tumor are done.[24]

In a patient who experiences some of the undesirable aftereffects of breast reconstruction, a physical therapist may be able to improve results with a technique called *myofascial stretching* or *myofascial release*. This procedure, which aims to increase pliability of the tissue, can be performed both prior to and after reconstruction. Dr. Ladizinsky has found the treatment to be very helpful for many of his patients. Myofascial stretching techniques are discussed in Chapter 10.

Reconstruction and Lymphedema

What about the effects of reconstruction on lymphedema? Dr. Ladizinsky reports that he does at times see swelling in the breast, trunk, or arm right after surgery, but he says it seems to be a short-term problem. So far, research does not show that reconstruction contributes to an increased incidence of lymphedema. However, there are variables in the standards for measuring lymphedema. For one thing, most studies researching the condition measure only arm lymphedema; that is, they do not include trunk or breast lymphedema. And although reconstruction may not cause a higher rate of lymphedema in the arm, most physical therapists who work with patients after breast reconstruction will tell you they see increased lymphedema in the trunk.

Furthermore, reconstruction using a patient's own tissue requires a great deal of surgery, which can contribute significantly to scar tissue, which in turn increases the chance of contracting lymphedema. Scar tissue creates an obstacle for lymph flow, particularly in the superficial lymph channels (those lying near the skin's surface). Women who have had this type of reconstructive surgery may notice some puffiness above or around their scars, or on the side of their trunk below the armpit area, or even in the reconstructed breast. Bottom line: While the good news is that swelling in the arm does not seem to be increased by reconstruction, there may be some increased swelling in the trunk.

Other Potential Complications after Reconstruction

As a side note, another concern with reconstruction procedures that use a patient's own muscle tissue is that the area from where the tissue has been removed inevitably suffers some weakness. This can contribute to muscular imbalances that may lead to pain and dysfunction. Instruction in posture, breathing, and exercise should be given to all patients after reconstruction to help them develop better muscle balance and strength, especially those who have undergone a TRAM flap or latissimus flap.

Furthermore, breast reconstruction can cause restrictions in mobility, discomfort, and numbness. These changes result from damage to the nerves in the armpit and scar tissue caused during surgery. Numbness in the armpit area occurs in *all* surgeries that involve axillary lymph node dissection and is often a symptom that bothers women more than scar tissue or swelling. The numbness can extend down the arm halfway to the elbow, and along the trunk below the armpit. Women describe feeling as if the area were bulkier or fatter than it actually is—as if there were a football under their armpit, or a wad of cotton stuffed against the side of their chest. It is similar to going to the dentist and receiving an anesthetic; it feels as if you have a fat lip, but when you look in the mirror you see it is not really swollen. The size of the area that feels numb decreases over time, but some women are left with a small area that never regains normal sensation.

If you are considering breast reconstruction, consult a plastic surgeon to discuss your options. Ask to see photos of both successful and less successful outcomes. Speak to other women who have undergone the various procedures. Ask them if they would work again with the same plastic surgeon. In her book *After Breast Cancer* Hester Hill Schnipper lists some good questions to ask other women about their overall satisfaction with the results of their reconstructive surgery, the recovery period, any problems they had, and whether they would make the same choice again. Schnipper writes, "The only good reason for breast reconstruction is because YOU want the surgery and YOU believe you will feel more whole."[28]

For breast cancer patients, a plastic surgeon's most common role is to perform breast reconstruction or revision, but in Sweden plastic surgeons actually treat certain cases of lymphedema using liposuction. Studies report that some patients with long-standing, pronounced lymphedema have demonstrated improvement after liposuction, but they must wear compression garments twenty-four hours a day for the rest of their lives to maintain the reduction in swelling.[29] Liposuction surgery is not used in the United States to treat lymphedema. Dr. Ladizinsky states a concern that while this approach maintains the larger lymphatic vessels, it destroys the smaller, superficial ones. Lymphedema therapists utilize superficial lymphatic channels in the treatment of lymphedema to bypass the deeper channels that have been compromised from breast cancer treatment.

Incidence of Lymphedema after Breast Cancer Treatment

Determining how often lymphedema occurs after breast cancer is difficult. It has been reported as occurring in as few as 5 percent of patients and as many as 70 percent. One study by the National Cancer Institute reported a 26 percent overall average incidence of lymphedema within two years after treatment for breast cancer. The incidence crept up to 45 percent fifteen or more years after treatment.[30] Much of the confusion arises from the fact that no real standards exist that define how to identify the condition. There are even discrepancies in how to measure it. Furthermore, the incidence of lymphedema after breast cancer varies tremendously depending on the types of treatment a patient has undergone. Here we'll attempt a little clarity.

The development of lymphedema after breast cancer is related to several things: the extent of lymph node dissection, the extent of breast surgery, and the amount of radiotherapy given.[14] Axillary lymph node dissection and the field of radiation (the area of the body that is irradiated) are the two greatest risk factors for lymphedema.[31,32] When breast-conservation surgery is done without radiotherapy or axillary node dissection, there is no increased incidence of lymphedema. Adding axillary node dissection increases the incidence, and adding axillary radiotherapy increases it even more.[30]

Lymph Node Removal and Lymphedema

Any surgical procedure that removes fewer lymph nodes will have the benefit of lowering the risk of lymphedema. In particular, sentinel lymph node biopsy (the removal and biopsy of only the lymph node or nodes located closest to the tumor) has been shown to dramatically decrease the incidence of lymphedema. One study demonstrated a 27 percent incidence of arm lymphedema in patients who had undergone axillary node dissection, compared to 2.6 percent in patients who had undergone sentinel node biopsy.[33] In addition to lowering the incidence of *arm* lymphedema, sentinel node biopsy also lowers the incidence of *breast* lymphedema.[34]

Dr. Gilbert, the surgeon who has been involved in researching SLNB, agrees that the incidence of lymphedema after the procedure is low. However, in women who do develop lymphedema following SLNB he sees more breast and trunk lymphedema than arm lymphedema, especially when extensive surgery has been performed on the upper outer quadrant of the breast. He says, "The incidence of lymphedema might actually be higher than is reported in the literature."

Breast lymphedema now seems to be more recognized than it was in the past. At the 2004 National Lymphedema Network convention, a presentation on breast lymphedema suggested that it occurs in 15–20 percent of breast cancer patients.[35]

Radiation and Lymphedema

Regardless of the type of breast surgery performed or the number of axillary lymph nodes removed, radiation is a significant contributor to an increased incidence of lymphedema.[36] An article in the *Journal of the National Cancer Institute* says, "A review of several studies reports lymphedema in approximately 41 percent of patients who underwent axillary radiation and surgery, compared with 17 percent of those receiving axillary surgery without radiation."[30]

The risk of lymphedema increases as the radiation field increases. Those at highest risk for lymphedema are patients who have had a full axillary lymph node dissection and who have also received radiation to the chest, axilla (armpit), and supraclavicular area (near the neck).[37] Dr. Nautiyal, the radiation oncologist, says he rarely sees arm lymphedema when he has treated only the breast with radiation, but when radiation includes the axilla, or if a patient has developed cellulitis (a spreading bacterial infection of the skin and the tissues immediately beneath the skin), he notices a great increase in the condition. It is very common to have some swelling in the breast with radiation. However, as common as it is, it frequently reduces on its own as women heal from the effects of radiation.

Radiation oncologists usually follow patients for only a limited period of time and may no longer be seeing them when lymphedema develops. In spite of this, most radiation oncologists are more aware than other doctors of a patient's potential to develop lymphedema and of the increased risk from radiation. Gwen's experience is that a high number of patients who come to her for lymphedema treatment are referred by radiation doctors. In fact, some radiation oncologists refer patients to her even *before* they begin radiotherapy, if the patient is going to have a large field of radiation and if the doctor feels there is a high risk of swelling.

Obesity and Lymphedema

It is important to devote some discussion to the apparent relationship between lymphedema and obesity. Multiple studies show that heavier women have a significantly higher risk of lymphedema.[37,38] A study done in 2001 by Dr. Allen Meek showed that breast cancer patients who developed lymphedema had an average body mass index of 29.5, whereas women who did not develop lymphedema had an average body mass index of 27.6. Body mass index (BMI) is defined as an individual's weight in kilograms divided by his or her height in meters squared. It is a measurement used by medical professionals to determine whether a person's weight-to-height ratio meets acceptable standards for good health. According to government guidelines, a person with a BMI of 30 or over is defined as obese, a person with a BMI of 25–29.9 is overweight, and a person with a BMI of 18.5–24.9 is normal. It is interesting to note that 67 percent of the women in Meek's study were above the normal BMI.[39]

A paper published in 2004 in the *American Journal of Surgery* studied the effects on the development of lymphedema of age, diabetes, smoking, hypertension, chemotherapy, radiotherapy, tamoxifen use, stage of cancer, body mass index, number of removed and metastatic lymph nodes, and total volume of wound drainage. Of all those potential risk factors, the researchers concluded, "Axillary radiotherapy and body mass index were found to increase the incidence of lymphedema."[14] These findings may present even more good reasons to work on getting those extra pounds off. If you're clinically overweight, losing some weight may help to reduce the effects of lymphedema. Diet and nutrition will be discussed further in Chapter 5, on prevention.

Lymphedema in Men

Although it happens only rarely, men can also develop breast cancer. When they do, they usually undergo the same treatment regimen as women: some combination of surgery, radiotherapy, and chemotherapy. Because breast cancer in men is so uncommon, it is often not detected until it has progressed to a later stage, when it usually requires more extensive treatment. As pointed out earlier, more extensive treatment increases the risk of developing lymphedema. This is true for men or women. Gwen has seen several men in her clinic who underwent breast cancer treatment. Two of them developed lymphedema after strenuous activity. They had never heard of the condition and were unaware of any precautions to follow. Their treatment was the same as it is for women who develop lymphedema.

No matter how overwhelmed a person may be by the diagnosis of cancer, no matter how dismayed a person may be at the choices that must be considered, it is important not to let a fear of lymphedema influence decisions about cancer treatment. People die from cancer, not lymphedema, and it is important to receive the treatment that will give you the very best outcome possible. That may put you at higher risk for lymphedema, but the benefits that come from survival far outweigh the risks of lymphedema. Lymphedema can be effectively managed, and education is the key. Read on. In Chapter 5 you'll learn what you can do to try to prevent lymphedema, and in Part II you'll learn about the many things you can do to treat it.

2

SIGNS *and* SYMPTOMS
of LYMPHEDEMA

This chapter focuses on the earliest steps of dealing with lymphedema: recognizing it and obtaining a diagnosis.

What to Watch For

Although the primary symptom of lymphedema is usually considered to be swelling in the area affected by the cancer treatment, several other signs can indicate its initial onset. If you notice any of the signs listed below, or if you are simply concerned that you may develop lymphedema, call your oncologist or contact the National Lymphedema Network (see Resources). Even though women who have endured lymphedema for many years have achieved relief after treatment, the sooner the condition is treated, the better chance you have of reducing the swelling and maintaining elasticity of the skin.[1]

Signs to look for include the following:[2,3,4]

* A feeling of pressure, heaviness, or tightness in the arm.

* A sensation of fullness or swelling, which can often be present even before swelling can be seen. Excess fluid in the body's tissues is not visible until it reaches 30 percent above normal. Also, 50 percent of people diagnosed with arm lymphedema report that the first symptom was a feeling of

heaviness or fullness in the arm, even before they saw any swelling.

* Puffiness, swelling, or any increase in the size of the limb or anywhere in the quadrant of the body that has undergone surgery or radiotherapy (arm, armpit, breast, another part of the chest, or around the surgical scar).

* A pins-and-needles sensation in the limb.

* A feeling of heat in the arm or in the affected side of the body.

* Redness and inflammation (this may indicate infection, so see your doctor right away).

* Pitting: If you press the skin and hold it in for a moment, it does not bounce back when released.

* A "bursting" sensation in the limb.

* Aching in the limb, shoulder, or shoulder blade area.

* The inability to pinch a fold of skin on the top of one of the fingers (between the finger joints) or between the forefinger and thumb.

Again, if you notice any of these symptoms, we recommend that you take it as a warning sign that more fluid may be coming into the area, even if there is no visible swelling as of yet. Any of them may be a precursor to lymphedema (sometimes referred to as *latent lymphedema*). Pay attention to how your body is feeling; in particular, monitor the response of your body to various activities. And if you suspect that lymphedema may be developing, stop whatever you are doing and take a moment to see if you can help the fluid drain out of the area. Do this by elevating your arm, drinking some water, and loosening any constricting clothing. Also try breathing deeply into the diaphragm, a technique described in Chapter 7. These are all easy steps you can take immediately. You'll find more detailed information about relieving fluid buildup in the chapters on treatment, located in Part II of the book. Of course, actual swelling is a sign that you probably have already developed lymphedema; in that case, in addition to following the simple steps outlined above, you need to seek more formal treatment.

Remember from Chapter 1 that there is no way to predict if, when, or precisely where you may develop lymphedema. It can start immediately after surgery for breast cancer or much later. It is not unusual for lymphedema to develop long after you have finished having regular and frequent appointments with the surgeons and oncologists who treated your cancer. Medical oncologist Stephen Chandler tells of one patient who didn't have lymphedema for many years after undergoing a lymph node dissection. He says, "She came to me following a powerful winter storm when she developed swelling after lifting bales of hay for her farm animals." Although the condition can come on at any time after treatment for cancer, Dr. Chandler commonly sees women developing lymphedema four to six months after treatment. He encourages patients to pay attention to changes in their bodies and adds that it is often up to the patient to notice when help may be needed.

Pain and Lymphedema

You may read that lymphedema is generally not painful, and for many people that is true. However, many lymphedema sufferers do experience significant discomfort, especially as fluid first comes into the affected area. The fluid exerts pressure against the tissue cells, which can create great discomfort. Sometimes the fluid applies pressure against the scar tissue on the breast or on the side of the trunk where the postsurgical drain tubes were located. Fluid can also distend the superficial tissue and the skin. Often, after a period of time—anywhere from a few days to several weeks—the tissue adapts and the discomfort decreases, in much the same way it would during pregnancy or after weight gain.

Lymphedema also makes the affected arm heavier and may even alter how it is used, both of which can stress the shoulder and the neck and thus contribute to pain. Consider the increased stress to the shoulders and neck of a woman who has very large, heavy breasts; lymphedema can affect the body in much the same way. For some, lymphedema can exacerbate preexisiting conditions such as tendonitis, bursitis, or arthritis, again because of the increased pressure or weight of the arm. In most cases, the discomfort can be reduced or eliminated with proper treatment of the lymphedema and of the condition it may have aggravated.

Finally, lymphedema can have huge psychological, social, and emotional effects. If the swelling is great enough, it can't be hidden. In fact, a swollen arm is far more visible than the loss of a breast.[5] This topic will be addressed in more detail in Chapter 19, on emotions and lymphedema.

Diagnosing Lymphedema

In most cases, a diagnosis of lymphedema can be easily made by your doctor—usually by your medical or radiation oncologist, but possibly by your primary care provider or surgeon. Your oncologist will most likely be more familiar with the condition than a family practitioner will; furthermore, he or she is familiar with the cancer treatment you've had.

The doctor will take a medical history and conduct a thorough physical examination. Depending on the circumstances, he or she may want to test to make sure there has been no recurrence of cancer, particularly if there's nothing you can point to that caused the swelling—for example, if you didn't do any harder than normal activity like shoveling snow or lifting bales of hay, or the weather hasn't turned hot, or you haven't taken a plane flight. If a recurrence of cancer has been ruled out and you have swelling in the area of the body affected by breast cancer, you are most likely experiencing lymphedema.

The International Society of Lymphology has categorized lymphedema into the following three levels:[6]

In Grade 1, pressure on the skin of the swollen area leaves an indentation that takes some time to disappear, as described in the list of symptoms. This is referred to as *pitting edema*. Sometimes the swelling can be reduced by elevating the limb for a few hours. There is little or no fibrosis (hardening) at this stage, so it is usually reversible.

In Grade 2, pressure on the swollen area does not leave a pit, and the swelling is not reduced very much by elevation. If the condition is left untreated the tissue in the limb gradually hardens and becomes fibrotic.

In Grade 3, often called *elephantiasis*, there may be gross changes to the skin in the affected area, including protrusion and bulging. Fluid may leak through the skin's surface, especially if there is a cut or sore. Grade 3 occurs almost exclusively in the legs, after progressive, long-term, and untreated lymphedema. Although the condition will respond to treatment at this stage, it is rarely reversible.

Some high-tech diagnostic tests, such as lymphoscintigraphy, MRI, and CT scan—all of which can accurately visualize the lymphatics—can confirm the diagnosis, but they are expensive and are rarely necessary to make the diagnosis of lymphedema after breast cancer. Such tests can be useful in a research situation, but they are not indicated for the majority of patients.

Some patients may be interested in seeing a doctor who specializes in lymphology. However, finding one can be difficult, since there are not many and they mostly practice in large medical teaching centers. If you want to find a lymphology specialist, contact the National Lymphedema Network (see Resources). It is important to keep in mind that your oncologist will most likely be able to accurately diagnose lymphedema; therefore, a referral to a lymphology specialist is rarely necessary. At the same time, although most physicians are familiar with lymphedema, they may be less aware of effective treatment options for it, so it would be helpful to ask your doctor for a referral to a lymphedema therapist if he or she does not suggest it. If you do not have any visible swelling but have simply noticed some of the warning signs, it would still be a good idea to ask your doctor for a referral to a lymphedema therapist who may be able to assess your symptoms and help design a program specific to your needs with a focus on prevention.

Take Lymphedema Seriously

Lymphedema may worsen with time if it is left untreated. It can become disabling by stiffening the joints or making the limbs heavy and cumbersome, and it may cause significant cosmetic deformities. Other serious effects include skin changes and fibrosis, plus, of course, the discomfort of having a swollen arm, breast, or torso.

An even greater concern is the potential for complications such as lymphangitis (a bacterial infection of the lymphatic system) or cellulitis (infection of the skin and the tissues just beneath the skin). Although it does not occur often, an infection in the area affected by lymphedema can become life-threatening since there are a decreased number of lymph nodes to stop a localized infection from turning very rapidly into a systemic one. An even less common—but more life-threatening—potential complication is lymphangiosarcoma, a very rare and aggressive type of cancer that can occur in patients with long-term, untreated lymphedema (existing for eight to ten years).[7] The good news is that because awareness is increasing in the medical community about lymphedema and its treatment, rarely will the condition ever reach the stage where such serious complications develop. Infections are treated early and aggressively, and treatment for lymphedema is increasingly available.

Though there are many things you can do to try to prevent the onset of lymphedema (see Chapter 5), if you have had surgery and radiotherapy to the lymph nodes you are considered vulnerable. It is important to know and to watch for the symptoms and, if you suspect you are experiencing some of them, to contact your doctor right away. Again, we wish to stress that if you do have lymphedema, the sooner you begin treatment and learn how to manage it, the better results you will have.

3

the LYMPHATIC SYSTEM

To understand lymphedema it is useful to first understand the normal lymphatic system. This short chapter will help you do that. (As mentioned in Chapter 1, however, your ability to *treat* lymphedema does not depend on you having an in-depth understanding of the lymphatic system.)

The lymphatic system has several important functions:

* ❋ It maintains fluid balance in the body by collecting excess fluid that is not absorbed by the blood capillaries.

* ❋ It removes proteins, waste products, bacteria, viruses, and other impurities from the tissues throughout the body.

* ❋ It participates in creating antibodies, proteins that are custom designed to fight infection and foreign invaders.

This list briefly summarizes *what* the lymphatic system does. Now let's examine *how* it does what it does.

Lymphatic Vessels

Remember from the first chapter that the lymphatic system is a part of the body's circulatory system. As such, it is composed of lymphatic vessels. The lymphatic vessels begin as microscopic, fingerlike capillaries situated in the spaces between cells (called *interstitial tissue* or *interstitial spaces*). Each lymphatic capillary has a "front gate" of sorts called an *initial lymph vessel* (remember that term; we'll return to it in a moment). It may help to think of a tissue's cells as marbles in a jar. The interstitial space is the space between the marbles; interstitial fluid fills that space.

Now we turn to the blood system. Oxygen- and nutrient-rich blood flows from the heart through the arteries to the blood capillaries. Blood capillaries differ from lymphatic capillaries. They are the microscopic blood vessels where arteries connect with veins. The "artery side" of a blood capillary is called the *arterial capillary*. Arterial capillaries deliver fluid and nutrients into the interstitial spaces and to the tissue cells. About 90 percent of the interstitial fluid is reabsorbed by the venous capillaries (the "vein side" of the blood capillaries) and rejoined with the blood, which is now depleted of oxygen and nutrients and which flows through the veins back to the heart.

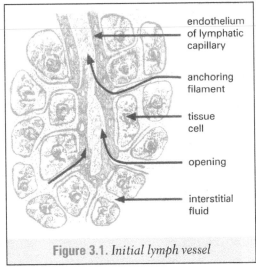

endothelium
of lymphatic
capillary

anchoring
filament

tissue
cell

opening

interstitial
fluid

Figure 3.1. *Initial lymph vessel*

Here's where the lymphatic system enters the picture. The initial lymph vessels absorb the remaining 10 percent of fluid left behind in the interstitial spaces, along with protein molecules, bacteria, viruses, and other waste products that are too large for the blood capillaries to absorb.

How Does Fluid Get into the Lymphatic System?

The initial lymph vessels have a slightly larger diameter than blood capillaries. They also have a structure that permits fluid to flow into them (see Figure 3.1). When the pressure is greater in the interstitial fluid than in the initial lymph vessel, the cell flaps of the vessel separate slightly, like the opening of a one-way valve , and fluid enters. As the vessel fills, the tissue pressure decreases and the valve closes. Once the interstitial fluid enters the vessel, it is called *lymph* or *lymph fluid*.[1]

What Happens Once the Fluid Is in the Lymph Vessels?

Think of the initial lymph vessel as the structure that opens the door to the lymph system, and the lymphatic capillary as the tiny vessel that carries fluid from that front door to the larger lymph vessel. Lymphatic capillaries gradually join together into bigger vessels called *collecting vessels*, which in turn become progressively larger as they converge and approach the lymph nodes. After flowing through the lymph capillaries and larger lymph vessels and being filtered through the lymph nodes, the lymph eventually drains into either the *thoracic duct*, which is the main lymphatic vessel in the torso, or the *right lymphatic duct* (see Figure 3.2). Over two-thirds of the body's lymph drains into the thoracic duct; the rest drains into the right lymphatic duct.

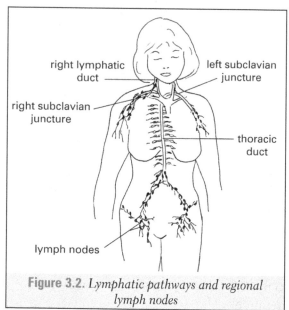

Figure 3.2. *Lymphatic pathways and regional lymph nodes*

From these two ducts, lymph fluid is rejoined with the blood at the left and right *subclavian junctures*, located in the lower neck. (*Subclavian* means "beneath the collarbone.") The left subclavian juncture is where the thoracic duct empties lymph fluid into the left subclavian vein, and the right subclavian juncture is where the right lymphatic duct empties lymph fluid into the right subclavian vein. The left and right subclavian veins converge with other large veins to form the even larger vein known as the *superior vena cava*, which flows into the heart.

How Does Lymph Fluid Move?

Lymph fluid is moved through the system of vessels and nodes by several driving forces—some within the lymphatic system and some outside it. Within the lymphatic system, fluid is transported by the following two actions:

1. Random contractions of the smooth-muscle wall of the lymph vessel, which occur six to seven times a minute. Valves located inside the collecting vessels allow lymph to flow in only one direction.

2. A stretch reflex of the *lymph angion*, the segment of each collecting vessel that lies between two valves (see Figure 3.3). When one angion fills, it stretches the nerves encircling it, causing a contraction, which moves the fluid to the next angion, causing that one to stretch and then contract, and so on.

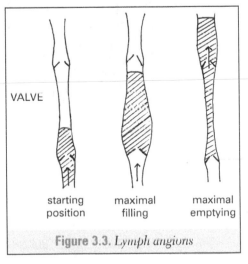

VALVE

starting position   maximal filling   maximal emptying

Figure 3.3. *Lymph angions*

Apart from the lymph system, other actions that influence the lymph vessels are:

* the pumping of the arterial system

* the pumping action of the muscles (see Figure 3.4)

* abdominal breathing, which causes a change in pressure within the chest cavity, stimulating the central thoracic duct

* peristalsis (the wavelike muscular contractions of the intestines)

* manual lymphatic massage

Because all these events affect the lymph vessels, they also present ways for you to take action to improve the efficiency of your

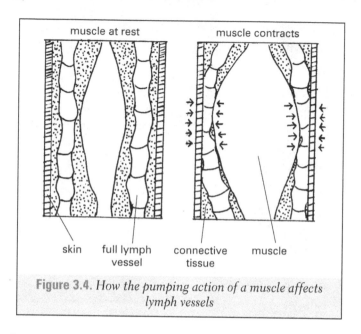

muscle at rest   muscle contracts

skin   full lymph   connective   muscle
       vessel   tissue

Figure 3.4. *How the pumping action of a muscle affects lymph vessels*

lymph system and thus to treat your lymphedema. We will look at some of these treatment options in Part II of the book.

Lymph Nodes

Lymph nodes are small, kidney-bean-shaped structures arranged in groups or chains along the lymphatic vessels. Between five hundred and a thousand of them are scattered throughout the body, but they are most heavily concentrated in the axilla (armpit area), groin, mammary glands, and neck. Lymph flows into the lymph node from the *afferent* (inflowing) lymph vessels, where it is filtered to capture and break down any foreign material or cellular debris (see Figure 3.5). The cleansed lymph travels out of the node in the *efferent* (outflowing) vessels.

The lymph nodes have two main functions. First, as already mentioned, they filter the lymph, destroying and removing dead cells, waste materials, protein molecules, bacteria, and viruses. These actions clean and fortify the lymph so it is ready to be returned to the blood. Second, lymph nodes produce and house *lymphocytes*, white blood cells that fight infection by in turn producing the proteins known as antibodies, which combat foreign invaders such as bacteria and viruses.[2] When an infection occurs somewhere in the body, the lymphocytes housed in nearby lymph nodes are triggered to multiply to battle the problem. Then, when infection disappears, most of the newly created lymphocytes die. But a few remain in case they're called into action for a problem later on. Our lymphatic system works to keep us healthy all the time, even when we are unaware of our need for its services.

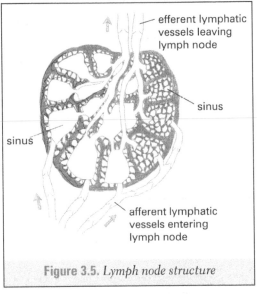

Figure 3.5. *Lymph node structure*

(efferent lymphatic vessels leaving lymph node; sinus; sinus; afferent lymphatic vessels entering lymph node)

The lymph nodes do not regenerate when they are removed or if they are damaged by radiotherapy. In other words, lymph nodes cannot repair themselves. While this may sound discouraging to those who have undergone a lymph node dissection or radiation, it is important to remember that breast cancer treatment affects only a very small percentage of lymph nodes, and that the system has some ability to compensate. In Part II of the book we'll discuss effective treatments to help stimulate the lymph system.

Watersheds

Watersheds are invisible boundaries that separate the different areas of lymph drainage within the body. Think of them as similar to the watersheds that exist on the tops of mountains: Water flows in one direction on one side of a mountain's watershed and in the opposite direction on the other side. (One patient referred to the watershed dividing the right side of her body from the left as the Continental Divide.) In this section we describe the body's main watersheds; there are more than the ones discussed here.

The body is divided by three main watersheds, a vertical one and two horizontal ones (see Figure 3.6). We will refer to each resulting area as a lymph *quadrant*. Although the term *quadrant* usually refers to one-fourth of something, medical professionals loosely use the word to describe an area of lymphatic drainage in the body

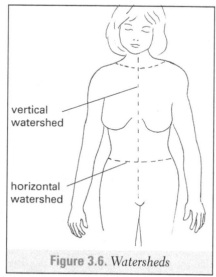

vertical watershed

horizontal watershed

Figure 3.6. *Watersheds*

(even though there are more than four such areas). Lymph vessels in each quadrant drain into a bed of regional lymph nodes; for example, lymph vessels in the area of the chest, back, and arm drain into the lymph nodes in the axilla (armpit) on either the right or the left side of the body. Small lymphatic vessels cross the watersheds and can transport lymph from one quadrant to another. Under normal circumstances, these lymphatic capillaries remain mostly inactive; however,

they are activated and become critical when the lymph system in one quadrant is not functioning well, such as following breast cancer treatment.

Having a general understanding of the lymphatic system's quadrants is important when working with the drainage techniques used to move fluid in lymphedema treatment. These techniques redirect fluid from a compromised quadrant to a healthy adjacent quadrant, where the fluid can be drained and filtered.[3] We will discuss the quadrants in more detail in the chapters on treating lymphedema.

The lymphatic system is both fragile and flexible. Though treatment for breast cancer may alter how well yours works, to a great degree you can take over for it to ensure your comfort and good health. You'll learn what you can do in later chapters.

4

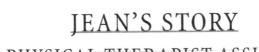

JEAN'S STORY
a PHYSICAL THERAPIST ASSISTANT
DEALS *with* LYMPHEDEMA

Jean and I first met over five years ago, at the center where she was
an assistant in the treatment of patients with lymphedema. She was
sixty-one then, short, round-faced, and square of build. Her com-
plexion was smooth and her smile brisk and ready. She worked at the
same facility where, several years earlier, she had been diagnosed
with breast cancer and had undergone a lumpectomy. Today Jean is
retired, but after her cancer treatment she put off initial plans to re-
tire because "the chance to work with lymphedema patients was too
interesting."

Jean's problems with lymphedema started about two years after
she completed chemotherapy and radiotherapy. She did some heavy
work one day while helping her daughter move, and afterward she
took a very hot bath. She emerged from the tub with a swollen arm.
When I first met her, the arm with the lymphedema was noticeably
larger than the other. She pressed her fingers into the underside of
her forearm. When she removed them, four deep crescents were left
behind. "I guess I need to bandage for a couple of days," she said.
(Bandaging is discussed in Chapter 12.)

Jean's life seemed to explode around the time she had cancer.
When she was halfway through her chemotherapy treatment, her
husband left her. "I just sort of fell apart," she told me with ironic

humor. "Everything happened at once: moving from the house we'd lived in for twenty years, the cancer, and my husband leaving." She chuckled. "You can get a lot of personal growth accomplished when all that happens."

She responded gamely to the crises she'd been handed. "I had every opportunity to fix what was broken," she said. "I worked in health care. And did I put the system to use!" She laughed. "I went to all kinds of counselors. I thought that since I'd always been the type to hold everything in, maybe it could have caused my cancer, and I wanted to learn not to hold *anything* in anymore. I just didn't have time to die. I wanted to see my grandchild. I had too much to do. I always wanted to square dance, so I took lessons, even though I didn't have a husband to do it with. And I had a wonderful time."

Jean and her husband eventually started dating again. She said, "By then I had stuff pretty much together, I mean, about the cancer and the loneliness without him. He was living across town but spending most of his time with me. I knew I wanted someone in my life, and I began to realize I didn't want to go on forever like we were, so one night I told him, 'Either you come home or I want a divorce, and I don't think I'm going to want to see you again.' I wasn't mad. I wasn't trying to hold on to him or to anyone. I just wanted to get on with my life." Grinning, she said, "He came home." They're still together several years later.

Jean is philosophical about her health. When we first met she told me, "I *hate* to be called a cancer survivor, because that implies I am a victim of cancer. I'm not a victim. I just had cancer, that's all. I want to get on with my life. I want to *do* something about it, not *think* about it. To me, working with lymphedema treatment is doing something.... I still have some life. I'd love to be part of a lymphedema clinic for low-income women who can't afford treatments. I could show them how to bandage and how to take care of themselves, maybe even teach them to team up and to massage each other."

She also made some astute observations about how well patients fared when they followed the self-help treatments taught to them at her clinic. "I noticed that our patients who do the exercises, who do the self-massages, who get out and live life, who walk, swim, ride bikes—they are the ones who manage okay with lymphedema. It's the ones who are depressed, who don't finish their series of treatments, who sort of give up, they're the ones who really end up with trouble. We had one woman who was eighty years old when she came in for treatment. She'd had lymphedema for several years. She was so skeptical. She couldn't believe it would work, but she kept at it and the swelling in her arm came down and she quit hurting. A while back she wrote us a note. She was vacationing with her family in Kansas. Now *that's* what treatment can do if you let it."

Jean said that after she retired, her lymphedema "just gradually went away." She still bandages occasionally, particularly when she flies. "I flew to Japan a while ago, and even though I bandaged, my arm got painful, so I'm real careful with it now. I'm also cautious with hot tubs and doing too much exercise at one time. Otherwise, I'm real healthy." She chuckled and added, "Except I'd like to lose fifty pounds."

5

PREVENTING LYMPHEDEMA

It is not clearly understood why some people develop lymphedema no matter what precautions they take, yet others never develop it no matter what they do. As discussed in Chapter 1, surgery and radiotherapy compromise the lymphatic system and leave a person with a higher risk of developing lymphedema for the rest of her or his life. Although there are no scientifically backed guarantees promising you won't get the condition even if you follow all the precautions in the world, you can definitely *lower* your risk of getting it. This chapter discusses precautions you can take, habits you can adopt, and lifestyle choices you can make that are good common sense and can reduce your risk. You will find many of these recommendations in the National Lymphedema Network pamphlet *18 Steps for Preventing Lymphedema* (see Recommended Reading, located at the back of the book). If you already have lymphedema, the guidelines presented here will help you to manage it better.

Helpful Hints

We've said it before, but it bears repeating: Education is the key. The more we know, the better choices we can make. Being informed is worth the effort. For example, if you feel an episode of swelling coming on, you will be able to recognize it, have an idea of what may have contributed to it, and, most importantly, know something to do immediately to help yourself. The first steps are always to elevate your arm, loosen any constricting clothing, practice diaphragmatic breathing (see Chapter 7), and drink some water. These steps, as well as many others, are discussed in more detail in the chapters on treatment. For now, we will focus on offering other helpful hints to reduce stress to the lymphatic system and thereby reduce the chances of developing lymphedema.

Avoid Infection and Injury

This suggestion may seem obvious. After all, who wants infection or injury? Most of us spend our lives trying to keep away from them. But avoiding them if you're at risk for lymphedema is especially important. That's because an infection brings additional lymph fluid to the area, increasing the potential for an episode of swelling. Many women have reported that their lymphedema started with an infection.[1]

Any break in the skin in an area of your body that may be vulnerable to lymphedema can lead to infection. Bacteria are everywhere. We breathe them. We eat them. They cover our skin. Most of the time our bodies deal well with the exposure to bacteria. But individuals with damaged lymph nodes or whose lymph nodes have been removed have a decreased ability to fight off bacteria and the harm it can cause. Scratched, burned, or cut skin is at great risk for infection. If you do get a cut, scratch, or any other injury that causes an opening in the skin on a part of the body that is susceptible to lymphedema, wash it immediately, then apply an antibiotic ointment such as Bacitracin. (Some wound care specialists are no longer recommending Neosporin or triple antibiotics because many people have developed sensitivities to them.) We suggest carrying with you at all times a plastic bag containing an alcohol wipe, a single use of topical antibiotic, and a Band-Aid.

Next, keep a close eye on the area for the next few days to watch for any changes in the skin. If you notice any signs of infection—rash, itching, pain, warmth, redness, streaking of color, sudden swelling, hardness, or high fever—contact your physician. An infection in a part of the body that is vulnerable to lymphedema can move quickly and become serious in a matter of hours. Your doctor will most likely prescribe oral antibiotics immediately. Generally, antibiotics in the penicillin category, such as dicloxacillin and Keflex, are very effective, but your physician will decide which one is most likely to work for you.

Developing a safer lifestyle can make all the difference in avoiding infection. Start by learning to change little habits that might cause injury, for example:

* Shred cheese with your unaffected hand (do you know anybody who doesn't nick themselves shredding cheese?), use a food processor for the job, or buy cheese that is already shredded.

* Wear long-sleeved clothing or use insect repellent to avoid bug bites. There are good, safe repellents on the market that you can apply to your clothing and that will last through several washings. Look for them at specialty recreational-equipment stores or on the Internet.

* Wear gloves and long sleeves when you garden and do housework.

* Rather than cutting your cuticles, moisturize them with lotion and gently push them back. If you get manicures, be sure to advise the manicurist to do this as well.

* If you have blood drawn, have an IV, or are given a shot, ensure that your affected side is avoided.

* Avoid pet scratches. Animals' claws carry a lot of bacteria. Swelling will often develop or increase due to an infection caused by a cat scratch. Pet stores and veterinarians now carry inexpensive little plastic caps that can be glued onto the tips of your cat's claws. Your cat may protest, but they are harmless to her and can protect you from scratches.

* Some experts recommend carrying oral antibiotics if you are prone to infections and are planning to travel outside the U.S. in an area where limited medical care is available. People who have a history of multiple infections or cellulitis

are sometimes given antibiotics to carry with them at all times, even if they are not traveling far.

It may take concentration to develop and make a practice of living with safer habits. One patient who wanted to remove warts used an over-the-counter wart medication. Within days she had a dramatic increase in swelling, and her arm never returned to its "pre–wart removal" size.

Avoid Pressure on the Involved Extremity

If your lymphatic system is compromised it is important to avoid constricting it in places where it is vulnerable. Constriction can eventually cause swelling in the chest wall, shoulder, or arm. Avoid anything that puts pressure on the involved areas. This even means asking that your blood pressure be taken on your unaffected arm. If you've had cancer treatment on *both* sides, your doctor or nurse may be able to use your leg to take your blood pressure or to deliver injections, although it might be challenging to convince them to do it this way. If you can't get the nurse or doctor to take your blood pressure using your leg or to give you a shot there, choose the arm with the least amount of swelling or the side that has had less cancer treatment and monitor the arm closely for any adverse effects.

Wear jewelry and watches only on your unaffected arm. Even a loose bracelet or watch could potentially cause a problem if it is bumped or catches on something and causes a cut or scratch. Furthermore, resting your arm can cause the jewelry to press against the skin. Keep an eye on any rings that you wear on your affected side to make sure you can remove them. If your swelling becomes too great, you may need to have rings cut off your hand. A possible solution is to purchase rings with expandable bands, called "arthritis" rings.

Another culprit can be a purse strap; pressure applied from hanging it over the shoulder can cause a backup of lymph flow. Avoid carrying your purse on the shoulder of the affected side.

Avoid Constrictive Clothing

Be careful with tight wrist cuffs and sleeves, especially if you have already developed lymphedema. You may no longer be able to wear a favorite dress, blouse, or nightgown because it unnecessarily constricts the arm. Wear clothes and nightwear with loose wristbands and sleeves. The sleeves of pajamas and nightgowns can slide up while you sleep and cause an indentation on your arm that you aren't even aware of until the next morning.

Buy the Right Bra

Brassieres pose a whole set of things to think about. Though some women become much more relaxed about wearing a bra after breast cancer surgery, most still follow convention and choose to wear one. To increase your chances of avoiding lymphedema, a good-fitting bra is critical whether you have had a mastectomy or lumpectomy.

Fern Carness, MPH, R.N., is a certified fitter for mastectomy products. She says the most common problem she sees is women with poorly fitting bras. Most women are really not the size they think they are. According to Fern an ill-fitting bra does not provide enough support, rides up in the back, and can cause constriction around the trunk, over the top of the shoulder, or on the side of the trunk. Any of these problems can block lymph flow. She emphasizes that no single bra works for all women. The type of bra that is right for you depends on many things: your size, your shape, surgical interventions you've had, conditions such as scarring or swelling, and your personal preferences.

The *National Lymphedema Network Newsletter*, in an article containing guidelines about the use of brassieres, recommends that anyone who's had an axillary node dissection *never* use an under-wire bra.[2] The article maintains that the pressure of the wire prevents the drainage of fluid from the breast and chest wall to other, normal lymph quadrants. Fern does not completely agree with this assessment. She says if the bra fits well and the wire supports the breast properly, there should be no undue constriction. Again, she believes that problems with under-wire bras arise when they don't fit right. If you want to wear an under-wire bra be sure to have the fit evaluated by someone experienced in fitting. Also be sure to monitor your body's response; notice if you have any increased swelling in the breast or trunk after wearing one.

The best bras for lymphedema have wide, padded, adjustable straps, which lessen pressure to the collarbone area. They have wide side panels, which support and cover the area on the side of the chest. Some women who've undergone a mastectomy have extra tissue, called a "dog ear," below the armpit, left there by the surgeon in case the woman decides to have reconstruction. It often becomes a reservoir for lymph fluid. If you have swelling under the armpit—a wide-banded bra better supports that area. And if the wide band doesn't offer enough support, you can wear a small pad beneath it to provide extra compression. A good bra for lymphedmea will also have a wider band under the breasts to spread the support over a larger area.

No matter which style you choose, make sure your bra has no visible areas where it binds, rolls up, or folds over. If you see indentations on your body after you remove your bra, have someone review its fit. In fact, it's best to have a professional fitter help you with bra style and size before you make your purchase. But not everyone has access to a professional. If you don't, you can find good-fitting bras in a department store, following the guidelines outlined in this section.

While this list is not all inclusive, here are a few suggestions for lingerie products designed specifically for women who have been treated for breast cancer. Keep in mind that even if we recommend a bra, it still may not be a good fit for your shape or may no longer be available for sale. There are also new designs being developed all the time, and there may be even better bras on the market at the time you are searching for one. You can find the following bras in specialty shops that specifically sell products for women after breast cancer. Some department stores carry them, too.

Louisa Louisa. These undergarments, which we highly recommend, come in both traditional bra and tank-top styles. They are made of a blend of Lycra and cotton that provides light compression, and they feature pockets for a prosthesis or for the foam pads worn by some women who have breast lymphedema. Fern Carness recommends wearing the tank top for traveling because it provides gentle pressure throughout the trunk. It offers an under-breast support band that goes only partway around the trunk, so it doesn't constrict lymph flow. The side of the garment, beneath the armpit, is wide, to provide constant compression to the lateral trunk (under the arm).

Jodee. These bras are good for plus-size mastectomy or lumpectomy patients who have lymphedema. They feature a "snuggle band" under the breast that flares out at the bottom so the bra doesn't roll up on women with larger abdomens. The side panels are very wide and have a pocket into which a pad can be inserted to reduce trunk swelling under the arm. Each bra even comes with a pad.

Bellise. This is an excellent bra, developed by a lymphedema therapist, that has recently come on the market. It provides good compression around the trunk, has wide panels, is easily adjustable with both front and back closures, and contains lots of pockets for padding or a prosthesis. The down side is that it is very expensive—around $250 (in 2004). Insurance may not cover the entire cost.

Anita Medical Bra. This European-manufactured bra is good for the woman who has asymmetrical breasts, which can occur following removal of a large lump or following radiation. It is very accommodating in fit. It offers many of the same components as the Bellise but is less expensive (although still relatively pricey). It zips or hooks in the front, is molded, has adjustable Velcro shoulder straps, and comes with additional attachable pieces so the wearer can adjust the fit.

Sports bras. Some sports bras provide a good fit, are very comfortable, and do not bind in any area. You may want to choose one with a hook or zipper closure rather than a one-piece style that you pull over your head.

Whether you go to a specialty shop to see someone trained in the proper fitting of bras or go to a department store on your own, you will need to try on several bras to see how they fit. The guidelines suggested above should help you to find one that works well for you.

Avoid Vigorous Activity

Don't bring on muscle fatigue. If you work out, don't "go for the burn" in your affected arm—or anywhere in your body for that matter. Make sure that whatever you carry is not too heavy, particularly if you're carrying it with your arm fully extended, as you would a packed suitcase. Avoid making vigorous, repetitive movements against resistance with your affected arm—for example, rubbing, scrubbing, pushing, or pulling, as with a vacuum cleaner. Heavy housework involves many movements that can trigger lymphedema, so try to find someone to help with it. If you cannot convince other household members to do some of the heavy chores, or if it isn't financially feasible to pay someone else to do them, follow some simple precautions. If you have short-stretch bandages, wrap your arm before you start your chores, and keep it wrapped the whole time you're doing them. Wearing bandages while doing housework offers a dual benefit: Your house will be clean, and you will have taken a step to decrease the fluid in your arm. (Bandaging will be covered in a later chapter.)

Since for most of us some housework is inevitable, here are more ideas to reduce stress to your arm:

* Use your unaffected arm or both arms.

* Do only small amounts of housework at one time.

* Take frequent breaks.

* Make moderation your motto. Pace yourself.

* Adjust your priorities. Determine what is really important. After all, what price are you willing to pay (with increased swelling in your arm) to have a clean house? Fatigue, heat, and doing too much can all increase the blood flow to an area, creating more fluid in the tissue, which can overload an impaired lymphatic system.

Directly after surgery and treatment, *gradually* return to your previous activity level, and always monitor the response of your arm, breast, or trunk to what you're doing. You may want to measure the circumference of your affected arm and use this measurement as a baseline to help you to determine how well your condition is staying under control.

Exercise Care while Shaving

The most common recommendation for shaving the armpits after breast cancer surgery is to use an electric razor. It makes sense. But electric razors can pose problems as well. The area is often not smoothly shaped after axillary lymph node dissection, but instead has new dips, creases, crevices, and scar tissue. It can be hard with an electric razor to reach all the areas under the armpit, which may cause you to push harder while shaving. Nonelectric safety razors can nick, so you need to take care with them, too. You may want to use a mirror and to shave very slowly and carefully, whether you use an electric or nonelectric razor. The good news is that after surgery and radiotherapy, many women experience a decrease in the growth of underarm hair.

Avoid Heat

Avoid anything that will bring heat to an area troubled by lymphedema, including sunbathing, sunburn (use at least SPF 30 sunscreen), and heat-producing ointments like Bengay or Absorbine Jr. Try to stay out of the sun, but if you must be in the sun at least cover the skin of the involved areas. Even a suntan, which may look healthy, is hard on the skin because it tends to dry it out. Consider wearing long-sleeved clothing or clothing that has sun protection built into it. Columbia Sportswear makes some great lightweight, long-sleeved shirts of a fabric that has SPF 30 built into it. An Internet search may yield other sportswear manufacturers that make sun-protective clothing. When traveling, be sure to guard against sunburn through the windows of a car or plane.

Stay out of hot tubs and saunas; they are some of the pleasures that can trigger lymphedema. You may think that you would be able to enjoy the hot tub by holding your affected arm out of the water, but often the temperature of the water is so hot that it raises the temperature of the whole body, including the trunk on the affected side. A man who had undergone cancer surgery and radiotherapy ten years ago and had never experienced lymphedema was advised to use a Jacuzzi following a car accident. After several weeks of his using the hot tub, the swelling started.

Despite the suggestion to avoid hot tubs, we find that many people still use them. If you decide to try, reduce the temperature to less than 100°F, keep your arm out of the water, and stay in it preferably less than ten minutes. As with all activities, monitor your body's response afterward to see if any swelling has started. If there are no signs of swelling, perhaps you may be able to enjoy the tub at times, carefully following these guidelines.

Try to take lukewarm, not hot, baths or showers. Avoid applying a heating pad or a microwaveable rice bag to any part of the affected quadrant of the body. This means if you have a back strain that is unrelated to the breast cancer or treatment, use ice on it rather than heat. If you sustain an injury your doctor may suggest using heat on it. That is good advice for most people, but not for a person who has had her lymph system compromised. (It is still okay to use heat on other, uninvolved areas.)

Hot weather tends to cause more swelling. You may want to find a cool place to go—like an air-conditioned bedroom or a cool basement—when the temperature and humidity are at their highest. Plan your outdoor activities for cooler times of day, such as early mornings or evenings. When the weather is hot you will need to pace yourself and allow more time for rest. Other cultures located in warm climates have it figured out; businesses and shops in Mexico, for example, often close down during the hottest part of the day so everyone can take a siesta. An article in the *National Lymphedema Network Newsletter* suggests taking a cool shower when its hot outside.[3]

When it's moderately hot use compression bandages to keep the swelling down (see Chapter 12). But if it's *really* hot, bandages or compression garments can raise your body temperature to the point where they are no longer helping to reduce swelling. In that kind of heat, use compression garments in the mornings, when it is cooler, but take them off if they get too hot and uncomfortable.

Finally, drink lots of water. Doing so is especially critical in hot weather. To the general recommendation of eight to ten glasses of water a day, add another glass for every ten degrees the temperature rises over 80°F. Many of Gwen's patients report a direct correlation between lack of water intake and increased swelling.

Avoid Extended Use of Diuretics

Diuretics reduce fluid levels in the body, and they are often the first thing a doctor (especially a primary care physician) might think of when consulted about swelling. But in the case of lymphedema, diuretics are not helpful for the long term. In fact, they can worsen the condition. Diuretics do decrease the amount of fluid, but they don't do anything to break down the protein, bacteria, and waste products that remain. In lymphedema patients who use diuretics, once the fluid in the affected area is reduced, there is evidence that a much higher concentration of protein remains. The elevated concentration can cause the tissue to become fibrotic (hard) and thickened, leading to increased problems with fluid removal.[4,5,6,7] Diurectics can also dehydrate the rest of the body.

Some medical conditions require the use of diuretics. If your doctor prescibes a diuretic, ask why. If she or he is only trying to treat your lymphedema, ask for a referral to a lymphedema therapist. Of course, your doctor may prescribe a diuretic for any number of other conditions, such as too much fluid around the heart or lungs or excessive fluid retention in general. If so, taking it is probably a much higher priority than not taking it, even if it is not good for your lymphedema. It is important not to alter any prescribed medications without first consulting with your physician.

Keep Your Skin in Good Condition

Try to keep your skin clean, soft, and moisturized. For those with lymphedema, good skin care becomes critical. Dry skin provides portal entries for bacteria. Wash with a mild, hypoallergenic soap that does not dry the skin. After washing, towel off thoroughly. If your skin is fragile pat it dry rather than rubbing it. Suggested soaps for moisturization include Dove, Neutrogena, Aveeno, Basis, Tone, and Oil of Olay.

After bathing, immediately apply a moisturizing lotion, preferably one that has no fragrance, has a low pH, and contains alpha hydroxy, vitamin E, or aloe vera. Some examples are Eucerin, Lymphoderm, or Nivea. Lac-Hydrin 5 and Aquaphor are other excellent products that your radiotherapist may have recommended. There are many good moisturizers on the market. Keep in mind, however, that even the best products may cause irritation to sensitive skin; we recommend paying close attention to how your skin responds to any product. What may be great for one person could cause a skin reaction in another.

During the day apply a lighter moisturizer that will not get grease on your clothes. Use a heavier lotion at night. You do not need to apply moisturizer to areas that are prone to collecting moisture, such as the armpit, elbow crease, and under the breast; rather, these areas should be kept dry by applying cornstarch or powder.

Choose a Lightweight Prosthesis

The National Lymphedema Network pamphlet 18 *Steps for Preventing Lymphedema* recommends that if you have had a mastectomy and choose to wear a prosthesis, wear a lightweight one. A heavy prosthesis may apply too much pressure above the collarbone, increasing the risk of interrupting the lymphatic flow.

Some prostheses self-adhere to the chest wall. They still require wearing a bra for support, but the adhesive takes the pressure off the shoulder strap. Many women who use the self-adhering prostheses love them and find them easier to wear than other types. If you use an adhesive, check your skin to see if it causes any irritation.

Insurance will usually provide coverage for a basic prosthesis, but any special features, like adhesive, may cost more than the allowed amount. Still, you may find that the additional expense is worth the increased comfort.

Plan Ahead when You Travel

When you have lymphedema or are at risk for developing it, traveling can put a great stress on the lymphatic system. We encourage women not to let a fear of developing lymphedema after treatment for breast cancer stop them from traveling. Travel does, however, require planning ahead and the following of some precautionary measures.

We've mentioned heat as a culprit in bringing on lymphedema. This is something to think about when planning travel. If you're planning to go to a warm climate, consider traveling in the cooler season. Also be mindful of traveling to higher elevations; the decreased atmospheric pressure can cause swelling. Even the reduced cabin pressure in an airplane can put you at risk. Gwen recently had a patient with mild lymphedema who was planning a month-long trip to the mountains in Peru, where she would be at nine thousand feet elevation. Because the long flight and the high altitude put her at risk for more swelling, she needed to take great care to practice all the precautions and suggestions outlined in this section. She also needed to wear her compression sleeve during the day and her bandages at night and to do her self-massage and lymph-drainage exercises regularly. (These techniques are discussed in greater detail in the chapters on treatment.) By following this advice, the patient was able to successfully manage her lymphedema during the trip.

Plan your travel wardrobe with lymphedema in mind. Dr. Judith Casley-Smith, in an article titled "Tips for Travel," offers the following hints: Wear loose, comfortable clothing that is open around the neck so you can easily move around in it. Loose clothing will help you avoid constriction, and if swelling does develop your clothes will not be overly tight. Wear a bra that doesn't constrict. Wear a compression garment if you have one, or wear short stretch bandages (discussed in a later chapter).[8] If you already have lymphedema and are traveling long distances or for an extended period, using your regular garment or bandages alone may not be sufficient to manage the added stress to the lymphatic system brought on by traveling. In that case the bandages can be applied right over the compression garment for better support.[9] Or, as Dr. Casley-Smith suggests, use two compression garments; that is, wear a second garment (perhaps an older one or one that is more stretched out) over the first. That way, if in spite of your best efforts swelling starts and the compression becomes constrictive, the top layer can be removed and you will still have some support. There is more information in Chapter 12 about how to recognize excessive constriction when wearing bandages.

As we mentioned above, if you have a history of infections, speak with your doctor about filling a prescription for antibiotics to take with you when you travel, just in case.

And move. Wriggle. Squirm. No matter how you get to your destination, whether in a car, plane, or bus, sitting for hours is a sure way to promote swelling. (In a moment we'll describe some exercises you can do in your seat.) Consider traveling when the bus or airplane may be less full, so you can move around more easily. Stand up and move as often as you are allowed to. Dr. Casley-Smith recommends getting out of your seat whenever the "fasten seatbelt" sign is turned off. If you are traveling by car, take frequent rest breaks, get out of your car, stretch, guzzle water, and move around. And avoid packing the car with so much stuff that you don't have room to squirm or wriggle.

Even if your flight is booked tight, there's a whole list of moves you can do in your seat. Some overseas flights show exercise videos, but if yours doesn't here are some techniques to get you moving. Turn your head from side to side. Squeeze your shoulder blades together. Press your hands together in front of your body. Pull in your abdominal muscles and press your lower back into the seat, and then lift your legs, one at a time, marching in place. Roll your shoulders. Rotate your arms in and out, like you're turning doorknobs, and flex and rotate your wrists. Squeeze a small ball; clench and extend your fingers. Do a couple repetitions of each exercise every half hour or so.

Practice diaphragmatic (belly) breathing for at least five minutes every hour (see Chapter 7). Maintain good posture, which can be a challenge in those uncomfortable airplane seats. Stuff one of the airline's small pillows behind your back, or take along your own small pillow. In a later chapter you'll learn about self-lymphatic massage for the neck. Do some for a few minutes every hour. Elevate your arm if you can; prop it up on your companion's shoulder, on the next seat, or on the window sill.

While traveling, avoid caffeine and alcohol, and, again, drink lots of water. Food served on airplanes, especially those little packets of peanuts or pretzels, can be very salty, and salt causes the body to retain fluid. Consider bringing your own snacks.

When you get to your destination be careful about carrying heavy bags, especially with your arm extended straight down. Dr. Casley-Smith suggests taking a suitcase that's as small and light as possible. No one but you will care if you wear the same outfit more than once! Get a suitcase on wheels. Pack two smaller bags with less weight rather than one heavy one. Use the carts available in airports, or use a porter. Check your bags at the curb if that service is available. Don't swing your carry-on bag over your affected shoulder. Be careful when pulling your suitcase from the luggage carousel; use the uninvolved arm, or have someone else pull it off for you.

If you've been wearing a compression garment, leave it on for a few hours after you land. If your arm seems swollen, try to elevate it. Get to a cool place where you can rest or take a cool shower. Practice more of the lymph-draining and self-massage exercises, and be sure to drink *lots* of water.

Healthy Lifestyle Choices

This section discusses healthy lifestyle choices in general. If you have lymphedema a healthy lifestyle is more important than ever.

Maintain Your Ideal Weight

Most of us know that obesity is becoming an epidemic in the United States. A study published in the *Journal of the American Medical Association* shows that in the 1990s the proportion of people who are overweight skyrocketed in every state.[10] According to a pamphlet published by the American Institute of Cancer Research, being overweight increases the risk of cancer of the breast, colon, endometrium, gallbladder, and kidney. The pamphlet also says, "[o]besity can increase the risk of coronary heart disease, stroke, diabetes,

high blood pressure, gallbladder disease, sleep apnea, [and] os-
teoarthritis of the knees, hips and lower back."[11] Furthermore, there
is research that links obesity specifically to breast cancer. Adipose
tissue (fat) contains higher levels of certain kinds of hormones that
may increase the risk for breast cancer or its recurrence. Ninety years
of research has shown that what you eat is an important factor in the
development or prevention of disease.[12]

As we discussed in Chapter 1, obesity is also a risk factor for lymphedema. Excess body fat can be a special problem if you have an
impaired lymph system, making it more difficult for lymph fluid to
pass through tissue and into the lymph vessels. The Memorial
Sloan-Kettering Cancer Center reviewed 263 women who had been
treated for breast cancer in the 1970s. Two factors were found to be
most significant in the development of lymphedema: weight gain
and incidence of injury or infection to the arm.[13] At the 1998 American Cancer Society's lymphedema workshop, Dr. Allen Meek reported that lymphedema is more common in obese patients.[14] In
2003 and 2004 multiple studies reviewing risk factors for lymphedema found that body mass index and axillary radiotherapy were
the two largest factors.[15,16]

Overweight lymphedema patients who lose weight may not necessarily see a reduction in swelling; still, weight loss certainly removes a load from the lymphatic system. Furthermore, many people
find that *gaining* weight can bring on an episode of swelling. Another study at Memorial Sloan-Kettering reported, "We were surprised to learn that weight gain following a cancer diagnosis is an
especially high risk factor" for lymphedema.[17] Unfortunately, women
who take tamoxifen or other long-term cancer-prevention medications may be prone to weight gain and have a harder time losing
weight.

It is clear that maintaining an ideal body weight is important to
overall health and to preventing and managing lymphedema. We
suggest talking with your doctor about specific recommendations regarding your weight.

Follow a Healthful Eating Style

While there are no specific dietary guidelines for managing lymphedema or dietary factors in the development of the condition, we recommend the healthy eating style highlighted by the National Institutes of Health and the American Institiute of Cancer Research.[18,19] (We like to refer to a person's eating habits as an "eating style" rather than a "diet." A diet is something you go on today and off tomorrow. An eating style is simply how you eat.) Their suggestions include:

＊ Consume a wide variety of plant-based foods.

＊ Eat plenty of vegetables and fruits.

＊ Maintain a healthy weight and be physically active.

＊ Drink alcohol only in moderation.

＊ Select foods low in fat and salt.

＊ Prepare and store food safely.

＊ Do not use tobacco in any form.

That's a good summary of a healthful eating style. The following general principles offer a little more detail:[11,19]

＊ Eat at least five servings every day of fresh vegetables and fruits. A serving size equals a medium piece of fruit, half a cup of cooked or raw fruit or vegetables, six ounces of juice (without added sugars), or one cup of raw leafy greens. The best nutrition is found in fruits and veggies that are red, orange, or bright green, such as broccoli, spinach, carrots, tomatoes, and red peppers. Include garlic and onion in your daily diet. Blueberries and raspberries have high levels of antioxidants; include a serving of one of them on most days.

＊ Eat 100 percent whole grains, including brown rice, barley, rye, oats, and whole-wheat pasta and breads. Try to avoid white flour. Cooked whole-grain cereals such as oatmeal are better choices than some of the cold cereals, which are often made with white flour. Whole grains provide an abundance of fiber, vitamins, and minerals. Diets high in fiber have long been recognized for their role in preventing colon cancer and heart disease. It is recommended that adults consume twenty-five to thirty-five grams of fiber a day.[20] Finally, the antioxidants and other phytochemicals found in whole grains are thought to help prevent cancer.[21]

* Eat beans, peas, and other legumes. Get a moderate amount of your protein requirements from beans and bean products such as tofu and lentils. Soy products can be protective against breast cancer, but limit them to three to five servings per week.[22] Incorporate a variety of seeds, nuts, and fish in your diet, and deemphasize meats, poultry, and eggs. But be careful about completely eliminating meats; it is important to consume enough protein. Since lymphedema is a high-protein edema, it might seem logical to reduce your protein intake, but it is absolutely necessary that your body have sufficient protein. Eating too little protein will not reduce the protein content in the lymph fluid, but it will weaken the connective tissue and worsen the lymphedema.[23] Nuts, besides being good plant-based sources of protein, are also high in healthy fats and omega-3 fatty acids. The better nuts include almonds, walnuts, and hazlenuts.[22]

* Try to minimize the fat in your diet. High-fat diets have been associated with cancer of the colon and breast. The American Heart Association recommends that dietary fat make up no more than 25 to 30 percent of one's daily caloric intake. Keep in mind that some fats are essential to health. The fat in fish has been shown to enhance the breakdown of other forms of dietary fat and to lessen the blood's tendency to form clots. The recommendation is to eat fish twice a week.[22] Extra-virgin olive oil is better than many other vegetable oils. Try to avoid margarine, most of which contains very unhealthful trans fatty acids (in the form of partially hydrogenated vegetable oils).

* Consume one or two tablespoons of ground flaxseed daily. Flaxseed is a source of omega-3 fatty acids and fiber, both of which are known to have specific breast-protective qualities.[22] Add it to baked goods, cereal, smoothies, or yogurt.

* Whenever possible, eat foods in a natural rather than a processed form. For example, fresh vegetables have more food value than frozen vegetables, which have more food value than canned vegetables.

* Minimize your salt consumption. Salt can cause water retention.

* Minimize your intake of caffeine and alcohol. Excessive use of these beverages may contribute to fluid retention. (Here's a side note for women that is unrelated to lymphedema: Excessive caffeine and alcohol also lead to excretion of calcium from the body, which can contribute to osteoporosis.)[21]

* Increase water consumption. Contrary to what may seem reasonable with lymphedema, a condition characterized by an excess of fluid in the body, it is imperative to drink lots of water. The high-protein concentration of the tissue in the arm, breast, or trunk attracts fluid from elsewhere in the body. Taking in less water will not cause less fluid to go to your arm; it will simply deprive the rest of your body of needed water. Drinking lots of water also helps to flush your system of impurities. It is recommended that you drink at least eight to ten eight-ounce glasses of water per day, and more in hot weather. You will encounter this suggestion several times throughout the book. Not only is it a good measure for preventing lymphedema; it is also on the list of things to do if you first start to notice symptoms. Drink a couple of glasses of water immediately, and then make sure you stay at the recommended level of water intake daily.

* Pay attention to portion sizes. An explosion in the "super-size" mentality has contributed to our country's obesity

epidemic. Even if you are eating healthy food, too much of it will make you gain weight. To lose weight, you have to burn more calories than you consume. Pay attention to how much you are eating; look at the serving size on nutrition labels. Use a measuring cup to accurately determine what a serving size is. You will probably be surprised.

* Don't become too hungry. Most of us have a tendency to overeat when our brain registers the idea that we're hungry. It is better to eat a little before you get to that point. Foods high in dietary fiber—such as beans, peas, lentils, or raw vegetables and fruit—will help to fill you up. To avoid getting really hungry, some people find it easier to eat several smaller meals throughout the day rather than three large ones.

* Here's a piece of good news: Chocolate is good for you in small amounts. (You knew it all the time.) Eating chocolate two to three times a week can be both a treat and good for you. Chocolate has flavonoids, which are rich in antioxidants. Semisweet dark chocolate is better than milk chocolate for two reasons: It has the highest level of flavonoids, and it doesn't have added milk, which can increase the saturated-fat content. Note that it's the chocolate we're talking about here, not the other goodies that might come with it, like caramels, marshmallows, or sugars. These don't increase the flavonoid count, but they do add fat and calories.[24]

Let's take a look at the eating styles of two non-Western cultures. It turns out that a Mediterranean-style diet is not just tasty but healthy as well. The Mediterranean diet, which is called that because it is based on the traditional eating style of several cultures from the Mediterranean region, includes many of the dietary recommendations listed above. It emphasizes eating more root vegetables and green vegetables, fresh fruits, beans and legumes, fish, whole-grain breads, fiber, olive or canola oil, and eating less meat, butter, and cream. Dr. Miles Hassell, of the Providence Cancer Center, recommends the diet. He cites the four-year Lyons Diet Heart Study, which followed people who had been recently diagnosed with heart disease. The study compared a Mediterranean-style diet to a typical Western diet. The results were dramatic: Individuals who followed the Mediterranean diet had 72 percent fewer major cardiac events, 56 percent fewer deaths, and 61 percent fewer cancers than their counterparts eating a typical Western diet.[22] This eating style has been around a long time. It is surprising that more physicians aren't recommending it.

Studies also show that Asian cultures, whose members eat a lot of fish, fruits, and vegetables, have a lower rate of breast cancer. Scientists suspect that the lower rate of cancer has to do with the differences in diet, but the issue is still being researched. As one study puts it, "Further studies of the lifestyle and dietary habits of non-Western populations may help in understanding etiologic factors underlying breast cancer development."[25]

Here are some cookbooks that incorporate healthy and tasty recipes: *The Mediterranean Diet Cookbook,* by Nancy Harmon-Jenkins with Drs. Antonia and Dimitrios Trichopoulou; *The Breast Health Cookbook,* by Dr. Bob Arnot; and *The New American Diet* cookbook, by Sonja L. Connor, M.S., R.D., and Dr. William E. Connor. These are listed in the Recommended Reading section located at the back of the book. Many other cookbooks also contain excellent dietary advice. Check your local bookstore or library.

Exercise Regularly—But Don't Overdo It

Exercise needs to be incorporated into all lymphedema-therapy programs.[26] In addition to being good for your health in general, it is good for your lymphedema. The lymphatic system is stimulated by the pumping action of the blood vessels and of the muscles, so anything you can do to improve your circulatory system will also aid the lymphatic system.

But don't overdo it. Don't fatigue or overwork the muscles, which can cause an increase in lymph fluid and make lymphedema worse.[27] Normally, swimming, walking, and bike riding are very good exercises for persons with lymphedema. Drs. John and Judith

Casley-Smith found that scuba diving was another wonderful activity for the reduction of lymphedema, with the effects lasting as long as two days.[28] This is most likely because of the increased pressure the body is subjected to when it is underwater.

The four categories of exercise recommended for lymphedema patients are covered in greater detail later in the book. In summary they are

* aerobic exercise

* stretching

* strengthening and toning

* lymph-drainage exercises

No matter what type of exercise you choose, do only a small amount at first—just a few minutes if you haven't been a regular exerciser, and a bit more if you are used to exercising somewhat regularly. From there, *gradually* increase your level of exercise over time, using your arm, breast, and trunk as monitors of how much you can do. And watch the temperature. Don't exercise in the heat of the day, and be sure to protect yourself from the sun.

We'll discuss specific details regarding exercise in Chapter 16. For now remember that exercise is a critical component of a healing/wellness program.

Until more research has helped to pinpoint exactly which activities trigger lymphedema and which help to reduce it, we recommend that you take a practical, commonsense approach toward managing your condition. Lymphedema happens because a person's lymphatic system is compromised, and a compromised system can become overloaded and cause swelling. Be kind to yourself. Keep in mind that no matter how careful you are you may still get lymphedema. Guilt about how you got it won't help a bit. Regret about putting in that flower bed or taking that airplane trip or carrying that grandbaby won't turn back the clock—and it certainly won't fix anything. Life happens. We do the best we can; we do what we think is right.

If we're at risk for lymphedema our best bet is to pay attention to our bodies. If you notice an increase in swelling or symptoms, slow down, back away from the activity at hand, and take a moment to reflect. Then change what you were doing when the swelling occurred, and learn techniques that will keep you healthy. Finally, don't become obsessive. (Though we know if you're worried it may be hard not to obsess.) The point is to live even if you do have lymphedema. Attend to it; work its care into your daily habits so you can forget about it and can get back to living, working, and enjoying life.

Part II can help you achieve these goals. It provides a complete treatment plan, with detailed descriptions of self-help techniques.

part two

TREATING
LYMPHEDEMA

6

an INTRODUCTION *to* TREATMENT METHODS

Some cancer survivors may be able to prevent an episode of lymphedema. Others will need treatment. Part II outlines in detail a complete treatment regimen. This chapter opens the discussion by providing a brief history of treatment and an overview of current treatment methods.

A Brief History of Treatment

Until the past decade, there were limited treatment options available in the United States for people who developed lymphedema. Most women were told that nothing could be done for the condition and to just "live with it," or they were placed on a compression pump and given a special compression garment to wear.

This state of affairs is surprising, because treatment of the lymphatic system has been widely practiced in Europe for almost seventy years. Manual lymph drainage (MLD, a light massage technique that moves lymph from one part of the body to another) was first developed in the 1930s by the late Dr. Emil Vodder and Estrid Vodder, of Denmark.[1] Their pioneering techniques eventually became known as the Vodder method. The work in the 1970s and 1980s of German doctors Ethel and Michael Foeldi helped to validate the effectiveness of lymphatic massage in reducing lymphedema.[2,3] The Foeldis combined the Vodders' MLD techniques with bandaging, exercise, and skin care. They named their method *complete decongestive therapy (CDT)*, a term still widely used today. Over the decades the Foeldis have conducted extensive research and published many articles and books related to lymphedema, and the Foeldi Clinic, in Germany, is still highly respected for its training of lymphedema therapists from all over the world. As the Foeldis were working in Germany, Dr. Judith Casley-Smith and the late Dr. John Casley-Smith began their work in Australia. In 1982 they founded the Lymphoedema Association of Australia.

Guenther and Hildegard Wittlinger, longtime pupils of Emil Vodder, opened a lymphedema treatment clinic in Austria and founded two schools to train therapists in the Vodder method of manual lymph drainage: the Dr. Vodder Schule in Austria in 1971, and the Dr. Vodder School of North America in the 1990s, both of which are still operating. The Vodder technique remains the most widely practiced and most commonly taught method in North America.[4] In 1988 the nonprofit National Lymphedema Network was founded in San Francisco by Saskia R. J. Thiadens, R.N., with the goal of providing education and guidance to lymphedema patients and health-care professionals from around the country. Ms. Thiadens also opened one of the country's first lymphedema treatment clinics, in San Francisco.

Dr. Robert Lerner, another pioneer, brought the complete decongestive physiotherapy approach for lymphedema care to the United States from Europe in the late 1980s. He conducted a landmark study on one thousand patients with upper-extremity lymphedema whom he'd treated between 1989 and 1995. The results showed that a program combining lymphatic massage, bandaging, exercise, and skin care produced an average 62 percent reduction in the volume of fluid in the arm.[5] He presented his results to the International Society of Lymphology, which published a consensus document recognizing the four-pronged regimen as the best treatment approach for lymphedema.[6]

The results of Lerner's study were supported by one conducted in 1997 by Marvin Boris, M.D., and Bonnie B. Lasinski, P.T., which followed patients who adhered to the same four-faceted treatment program. The researchers reported an average 63 percent reduction in the volume of fluid in patients' arms. The study also showed that patients who were most compliant in their follow-up care were able to maintain their initial reduction in swelling and even to improve it.[7] And in 2003 Dr. Andrea Cheville, from the University of Pennsylvania, reported, "Complex decongestive physiotherapy (CDP) has emerged as the standard of care[,] combining compression bandaging, manual lymphatic drainage, exercise and skin care with extensive patient education." She concluded, "Case series collectively describing a mean 65 percent volume reduction in over 10,000 patients attest its efficacy."[8]

In 1998, lymphedema experts from all over the world met in New York City and as a group officially endorsed the protocol of lymphatic massage, bandaging, exercise, and skin care as the most effective way to treat the condition.[9] (We would agree with Andrea Cheville that patient education is a fifth important component of a comprehensive treatment program.) The group settled on an official name for the regimen: *decongestive lymphatic therapy*. However, you will most commonly still hear it referred to as complete decongestive therapy or CDT.

Awareness of lymphedema and how to treat it is gradually spreading throughout the American medical community due to the efforts of organizations such as the National Lymphedema Network, the Lymphology Association of North America, the Lymphatic Research Foundation, and the International Society of Lymphology. Because multiple programs in the United States and Canada train health practitioners to treat lymphedema, competency standards needed to be established. The Lymphology Association of North America (LANA) developed standards with input from experts in the field. It also administers a national exam for the certification of lymphedema therapists. An inpatient lymphedema clinic now exists in Olympia, Washington, to provide intensive treatment. You can find a list of lymphedema organizations, schools, clinics, and products in Resources, located at the back of the book.

General Principles of Treatment

To recap, then, the following are the basic components of a comprehensive lymphedema treatment program:

* Lymphatic massage

* Compression

* Exercise

* Skin care

* Education

We have emphasized the importance of education throughout this book. Skin care was addressed in Chapter 5. Later chapters go into detail about massage, compression, and exercise. You will learn how they work and how to incorporate them into your life.

Lymphedema treatment is designed to stimulate the intact lymph system, improve the drainage of lymph from the compromised quadrant, and prevent lymph from pooling. As we explained in the book's early chapters, lymph fluid continually moves through the body, and breast cancer treatment can damage the ability of the lymph system to adequately drain fluid from the quadrant of the body affected by the cancer. If more fluid comes into an area than is able to drain out because of an impaired lymphatic system, the fluid will pool. This is described as exceeding the transport capacity.

The initial phase of treatment is rather intensive, typically involving frequent visits to a lymphedema therapist for all components of the program. The goal in this phase is reduction of swelling. The length of time for the intensive phase can vary depending on the patient and condition but is usually two to four weeks. Once the swelling has stabilized a maintenance program can be followed, using the parts of treatment that most help the individual patient. There's no doubt, however, that the more consistent and thorough a patient is in following through with self-treatment, the more effective the management of the condition will be.

In light of how busy most people's lives are, we believe that they will want to spend the least amount of time possible to get their symptoms under control and manage the swelling. Furthermore, treating lymphedema is not like cooking: There's no recipe that will turn out exactly the same for everyone. To some degree it is trial and error. You use the response of the affected quadrant as a barometer to gauge which aspects of treatment are most helpful for you. What is presented here is not the "only way," simply one "recommended way." As medical oncologist Stephen Chandler says, "All of my patients who have sought help have been gratified [by this program] and have benefited in some way. Some people have time to devote to it and some don't; it is time-consuming. All who have had treatment for lymphedema have been pleased that someone knows how to help. The approaches women take to deal with lymphedema will benefit them for the rest of their lives."

Philosophies about and approaches to lymphedema treatment may vary somewhat, but the basic goals are always the same: to reroute the fluid from the side of the body that's impaired to an area of better drainage; to provide compression to the swollen area in order to prevent lymph fluid from pooling; and to use the muscles' pumping action to stimulate the lymph vessels. The following chapters combine Gwen's experience as a lymphedema therapist with a distillation of the work of experts worldwide.

Before we launch into a discussion of specific treatment techniques, there are some simple things you can do right now to help yourself: Elevate your arm, drink more water, and practice abdominal breathing.

Elevation—that is, using gravity to drain the fluid from the affected body part—in the early stages of an episode is sometimes effective.[10] This was one of the few suggestions doctors offered in the past, and as a result many people have gone to great lengths to keep their swollen limb up in the air. While we don't necessarily recommend tying your arm to a pulley on the bedroom ceiling (yes, some patients have tried that!) or walking around with your arm raised, we can offer other simple suggestions. Try placing your arm on pillows while in bed, putting your arm over the back of the couch while watching TV or reading, propping your arm up on the shoulder of the person sitting next to you, and (if possible) lying down during the day for short periods with your arm elevated higher than your heart. When you are in the car, you can rest your arm on the window ledge, as long as you keep your arm covered to avoid exposing it to the sun.

The second suggestion is easy: As recommended several times throughout the book, drink eight to ten glasses of water per day.

Finally, abdominal breathing (also called *diaphragmatic breathing* or *belly breathing*) is a useful way to stimulate the lymphatic system. How to do it is explained in the next chapter. Some of the self-help methods described later include abdominal breathing as part of their instructions, so we recommend learning this technique before moving on to other ones.

These three simple measures may help to decrease swelling, particularly during the early onset of lymphedema. (In later stages elevation may have little effect.) However, taking these steps should not be your only course of action. If your arm is swollen, seek help. In the chapters to come you will learn many very effective strategies, and you will learn how to find a qualified health practitioner who can help you. We suggest you earnestly try every technique we describe.

7

ABDOMINAL BREATHING

To live, we have to breathe; we don't have a choice about that. But *how* we breathe is something we can choose. Learning to breathe in a manner that moves the abdominal muscles is an easy way to create an ongoing gentle pumping action to the central lymphatic vessel in the chest cavity (the thoracic duct), and thus to stimulate the flow of lymph. When you inhale using your abdominal muscles the pressure in the chest cavity changes because the breath moves the diaphragm. Likewise, when you exhale using your abdominal muscles, the pressure changes once again. The alternating pressure acts like a pump on the thoracic duct, which runs upward through the chest cavity and drains into the venous system at the neck. If you learn to breathe this way all the time, not just during your lymphedema treatment sessions, you'll be gently pumping your lymphatic system throughout the day.

In addition to stimulating the lymphatic system, diaphragmatic (abdominal) breathing offers many other great benefits, such as increasing oxygen to tissue cells throughout the body, lowering heart rate, decreasing blood pressure, relaxing muscles, and creating a relaxation response. Alice Domar, assistant professor of medicine at Harvard Medical School and director of the Mind/Body Center for Women's Health, teaches deep breathing as a life skill. She has found that women who practice it are able to reduce hot flashes, reduce symptoms of PMS, and help with pain control and anxiety.[1] She recommends doing what she calls "minis": taking several slow,

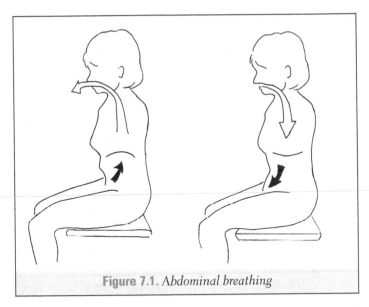

Figure 7.1. *Abdominal breathing*

mindful, deep breaths throughout the day, whenever you feel the need to promote more relaxation (or, for our purposes, to stimulate the lymphatic system).

Here's how the anatomy of belly breathing works. The diaphragm is a large sheet of muscle located just beneath the lungs, separating the lung cavity from the abdominal cavity. When it is relaxed it looks like a dome. As you inhale, the diaphragm contracts and pulls downward, creating a negative pressure, and the lower lobes of the lungs fill with air. At the same time, the diaphragm pushes on the abdominal cavity, and the belly expands outward to accommodate the extra air in the lungs. When you exhale, the diaphragm relaxes, returning to its dome position, forcing air out of the lungs, and flattening the belly (Figure 7.1). Watch how babies breathe. They naturally belly breathe. When a baby breathes in, its belly puffs out like a balloon. When it breathes out, its belly flattens.[2]

Notice that it is impossible for your diaphragm to move downward if your stomach muscles are tight. To get the most out of each breath, you need to relax your abdominal muscles. Unfortunately, starting at a young age most of us were trained to hold our stomachs in, which becomes more habitual as we grow older and have more belly to hold in. This habit has caused most of us to shut off our natural diaphragmatic breathing. It takes practice to undo that years-long habit and train ourselves to relax the belly and let the diaphragm drop down.

When you belly breathe, your breathing becomes deep and relaxed. It also becomes slower—since more oxygen comes in with each breath, you don't need as many breaths. Most people, rather than allowing their lungs to completely fill with air, breathe by moving only the upper parts of their chest and raising their shoulders. We fall into shallow breathing patterns for a variety of reasons: as a response to stress or pain, or due to respiratory problems, allergies, habit, or that ever-present belief that we need to hold our stomachs in. Many of us even hold our breath at times. To promote health, you want to provide your body with the most oxygen possible and help your lymphatics to pump efficiently. A smooth, even belly-breathing pattern is important.

Here's how to practice the skill.

How to Breathe Abdominally

First, concentrate on your breathing. Become aware of how you actually breathe. As essential as breathing is, most of us are never aware of our breathing patterns. To concentrate on it for a moment, sit in a straight-backed chair with your feet flat on the floor. Rest your hands gently against your abdomen. Without trying to change your breathing or force yourself to breathe in any particular way, just notice whether your belly is expanding or flattening as you breathe. You might find it easier to close your eyes while you focus on your next few breaths.

If you notice that your belly is expanding into your hands as you inhale, you are probably breathing with your diaphragm (at least in part). If your hands are still and your belly doesn't move much while you breathe, you are most likely breathing from your upper chest

The next step is to start practicing abdominal breathing.

Stay in the same upright position in the chair, and if you have a tight waistband or belt, now is a good time to loosen it. Take in a deep breath through your nose, and then exhale completely through your mouth, flattening your belly and squeezing out every last bit of air. Emptying the lungs completely and removing all the stale air from the bottom of the lungs automatically stimulates a diaphragmatic breath. Now, again breathe in through your nose, relax your stomach muscles, and notice how your belly expands. Allow the breath to start at the belly, gradually expand the ribs slightly, and finally come all the way up to gently lift the collarbones. Repeat the sequence. Let the air out through your mouth, making sure your belly flattens. Try another one or two breaths this way. (Some people prefer breathing in and out through the nose instead of inhaling by nose and exhaling by mouth. If that is easier for you, then do it that way. Allow yourself to breathe in whatever way is most comfortable for you.) If you get light-headed try to slow down your inhalation, and pause before breathing in again.

After the first couple of breaths, continue a gentle breathing pattern, inhaling through your nose and exhaling through your mouth, allowing your tummy to gently expand and contract. It is not necessary to take a giant breath—just one that goes to the bottom of your lungs while your chest remains still or slightly lifts. As Alice Domar points out, "Abdominal breathing does not mean that you don't take air into your upper chest; you do. But now you are also bringing air down in to the lower portion of your lungs by using your diaphragm to expand the entire chest cavity." It may help to keep your hands on your belly and try to gently push your abdomen into your hands as you inhale. Some people lie on their back and place a book on their belly. When you inhale try to make the book rise, and when you exhale try to lower it.

If using an image helps, picture a balloon in your lower stomach that inflates when you inhale and deflates when you exhale.

Finally, hearty laughter can be a great way to stimulate the diaphragm and help you breathe better. Most people have experienced a sore stomach and a more light-hearted mood after they have laughed long and hard, such as after viewing a funny show, watching a playing puppy, or listening to a comedian. Norman Cousins says, "Hearty laughter is a good way to jog internally without having to go outside." You will read more about Norman Cousins and the benefits of laughter in Chapter 21, "The Powers of Mind and Spirit."

Some Tips

Here are some suggestions for getting started (adapted from the workbook used in the Kaiser Permanente Managing Stress and Anxiety classes):[3]

* Start practicing with only four or five breaths, and slowly increase your practice time to one minute or longer. Practice several times a day.

* In the beginning, you might find it helpful to practice while lying down on the bed or floor. Bend your knees and place your feet comfortably apart.

* If you feel light-headed, dizzy, or anxious you may be breathing too deeply or too quickly. If that happens stop practicing for a moment and breathe normally until the symptoms pass. When you try again, slow down your breathing.

* Remember to relax the belly so the diaphragm can move downward.

* Be patient. At first this way of breathing may seem awkward; some people wonder how it could possibly be right.

As you practice and generally become more aware of your breathing, belly breathing becomes more natural and you may find yourself automatically doing it. It is a simple and effective way to stimulate the lymphatic system all day long.

8

LYMPHATIC MASSAGE

Lymphatic massage is a special form of very gentle massage that removes excess fluid and protein from an area affected by lymphedema and encourages the fluid to move into an area where it can drain away normally. The main physiological effects of lymphatic massage are to drain and cleanse the tissues, to cause a relaxation response by stimulating the parasympathetic part of the autonomic nervous system, and to relieve pain.[1]

It is important for lymphedema sufferers to receive massage treatments from someone who has been thoroughly trained in lymph drainage massage. Other types of massage, such as deep-tissue massage, can cause an *increase* in fluid to the area affected by lymphedema. Gwen tells of a patient who experienced pressure, heaviness, and aching in her arm eight years after breast cancer. She went for a deep-tissue massage and asked the massage therapist to focus on the arm because it had been bothering her. Within hours her arm started to swell. It is fine to get deep-tissue massage in the areas uninvolved in the treatment of breast cancer, but it is best to avoid any sort of heavy massage in the quadrant affected by cancer. Any therapist providing lymphatic massage must have a complete understanding of the dynamics of lymphedema and its treatment.[2,3] See Resources if you wish to find clinics and therapists with proper training.

The Principles of Lymphatic Massage

The term *manual lymph drainage* (MLD) was coined by Emil and Estrid Vodder to describe the specialized techniques used in lymphatic massage. Some practitioners refer to it as *lymphatic mobilization*. MLD starts with areas of the body that are *not* affected by lymphedema. The goal is to empty those areas first, clearing them to allow a place for the fluid to drain into. Since the neck is near the end of the lymph system—that is, where the lymph system joins the venous system just before the large veins enter the heart—the massage begins there. The neck area is massaged to clear it of fluid and to stimulate the lymph angions to contract. (Remember from Chapter 3 that lymph angions are the individual segments of the lymph vessels.) Research indicates that lymphatic massage of the neck area can stimulate activity in lymph angions located even as far away as the big toe![4]

Next, the therapist massages the uninvolved side of the trunk, gradually moves to the involved side, and finally massages the involved limb. Massage of a limb affected by lymphedema starts with the area closest to the trunk. First you massage the upper arm or upper leg, and then move down the arm toward the hand, or down the leg toward the foot. But the strokes always move in the direction of desired lymph flow (for example, toward the shoulder when massaging the arm). Massage of the abdominal area may be included to stimulate the deep lymphatic vessels. Throughout the massage, it can be helpful to practice the abdominal breathing technique described in Chapter 7. Rest your hands lightly on your belly so you can tell if your abdomen is expanding as you inhale.

The touches involve a special pressure/release stroke and are gentle, slow, rhythmical, repetitive, circular, and light. The pressure used should be just enough to cause a wrinkling of the skin; it should never cause redness or pain. Different types of strokes are used depending on which area is being massaged, the type of tissue, the integrity of the tissue, the size of the area, and so on. Although all lymphatic massage strokes employ a light pressure, a slightly firmer pressure is needed in areas that are fibrotic (hardened) or thickened. In more fragile areas, the pressure should be very light.

Different massage sequences are used depending upon the type of cancer and surgery, where the lymphedema is located, whether the patient has received radiotherapy, and whether one or both sides of the body are involved. Usually the massage takes forty-five minutes to an hour, but it can take longer if both the arms and the trunk are involved. The procedure should be very soothing. People often fall asleep during a session. Gwen typically suggests that patients practice abdominal breathing during the massage and visualize the fluid moving in the direction of the therapist's hands.

When Should You *Not* Have a Massage?

There are times when it is advisable not to receive lymphatic massage:[5]

* *If you have an infection in the area affected by lymphedema.* Signs of infection in the arm include redness, warmth to the touch, pain, and a sudden, unexplained increase in swelling. After an effective course of antibiotics, when the infection is gone, massage can be resumed. Some physicians will allow patients to resume compression (see Chapter 12) after several days on antibiotics and if the infection is clearly going away.

* *If you have congestive heart failure.* Lymphatic massage moves fluid out of the limb and through the body in the direction of the heart. A person with congestive heart failure already has too much fluid around the heart, so lymphatic massage could have life-threatening consequences. It may be permissible under some circumstances, but only with strict and close medical monitoring. Discuss your situation with your doctor and therapist.

* *If you are being treated for thrombosis or blood clots.* Lymphatic massage has the potential to dislodge clots, allowing them to move to the heart or lungs, where they could be fatal. Massage must be avoided if you are being treated for this condition.

❋ *If you have recently received radiation.* It is best to delay undergoing lymphatic massage because the skin will be quite fragile. In such cases it is possible to do some modified massage, avoiding areas of fragile skin until they are healed.

In the past it was thought that people with active cancer should not have lymphatic massage because it could move cancer cells to a new area, potentially spreading the cancer. However, this theory is now considered obsolete. Most doctors feel the risk of spreading cancer cells by mechanical measures such as massage is negligible and that having active cancer should not be a contraindication for lymphedema treatment. As all cases are different, discuss your situation with your doctor and therapist and decide what is best for you. If someone with terminal cancer has lymphedema, palliative care can often afford comfort and relieve pain. It certainly should be provided if the patient requests it.

Preparations for Treatment

To design an appropriate treatment and exercise program for you, your therapist will probably take a thorough medical history that includes your current symptoms. You may be questioned about blood pressure, thyroid problems, chronic inflammation, asthma, and other health issues that could affect treatment. The therapist will want to take precautions if you suffer from kidney disease, diabetes, hypertension, asthma, or arterial disease. After reviewing your medical history she or he may even decide that comprehensive lymphedema treatment should not be undertaken—for example, if there is a blood clot in the affected area or anywhere else in the body. In that case, parts of the self-treatment program can be taught—such as elevating the limb, belly breathing, and increasing fluid intake—but compression, massage, and exercise need to be avoided.

Self-Massage Techniques

Lymphatic massage done by a therapist is just one part of a total program to control lymphedema. You can also practice self-massage to maintain and promote the reduction in swelling. Indeed, self-massage is likely to become an integral part of your treatment program. We believe the work you can do for yourself offers long-term benefits and is an important supplement to treatment provided by a therapist. It gives you a way to more effectively control the lymphedema and empowers you to treat yourself immediately when a therapist is unavailable. If you notice your lymphedema increasing, as it might during hot weather or when you're traveling on an airplane, you can quickly take action to limit or eliminate a buildup of fluid.

As with MLD done by a therapist, when you massage yourself you begin with your neck and trunk before moving to the involved arm or breast. It can even be helpful to massage just the neck and trunk, because doing so clears the way and gives the limb a better chance of draining. In fact, trunk massage is so important that Gwen finds it best to emphasize it first so that patients do not, in their haste to reduce the swelling in their arm, move too fast to massaging the arm. If only the arm is massaged, the fluid will move to the top of the arm but then will flow right back into it. The trunk and neck must be cleared first to make room to receive the fluid.

Gwen suggests that patients perform self-massage before they apply compression bandages and do the exercises, both of which are described in later chapters.

General Guidelines

What we've described below is one possible self-massage routine; your therapist may suggest another. The important thing is to follow the sequence of first stimulating the neck, then the trunk, and finally the arm, and also to observe the other guidelines listed here. Again, it is important to work with a therapist who has been thoroughly trained in lymphedema treatment.

Make sure the area is free of oils, creams, or talcum powder so your hands don't simply slide over the skin.

Use flat fingers or the palm of your hand. The more contact your hand has with the skin, the more lymph vessels you stimulate. Do not push in with your fingertips. The massage requires two types of strokes: *stationary circles*, which are half-circle motions made in one spot, and *sweeps*, in which the skin is pushed gently in the direction in which you want the fluid to flow. In both cases, perform the strokes very slowly; each stroke should take at least one second to complete.

The pressure of your touch should be very, very light. Apply just enough pressure to cause the skin to move slightly. The skin may wrinkle in front of your hand or finger and/or spring back when you lift your hand. Release the pressure after each stroke, creating a repetitive, pressure-on/pressure-off pattern. The goal of the massage is to stimulate the lymph vessels to contract by moving or streching the skin, but always keep in mind that lymphatic massage should *never* cause pain or reddening of the skin.

Massage strokes on the arm should be directed toward the outside of the arm and then up toward the body. Visualize moving the fluid away from your hand and toward your heart.

Take deep abdominal breaths throughout your self-massage, inhaling through the nose and relaxing the abdomen as it fills with air, then exhaling through pursed lips as you pull in the stomach muscles, contracting the abdomen (see Chapter 7, "Abdominal Breathing").

<u>Self-Massage for Upper Extremities</u>

Start with an abdominal breathing exercise. Whenever stationary circles are recommended, they should be repeated twenty times. All sweep motions should be repeated five to seven times. Remember that all strokes should be slow and rhythmical, maintaining as much contact as possible between your palm or fingers and your skin. Review the material on watersheds in Chapter 3 so you will have a general understanding of where your vertical and horizontal watersheds are located. [The numbers of the steps below correspond with the numbers on Figure 8.2.]

1. Using stationary circles massage your neck in the hollow above both collarbones with your hands crossed (Figure 8.1). Or you can do one side at a time if that is easier for you. Make small, coin-sized circles, applying just enough

pressure to stretch the skin downward toward the heart and then
releasing it upward. The pressure
or skin stretch is applied in the
direction in which you want the
fluid to move.

2. Place your hand on the side of
   your trunk *on the uninvolved side,*
   just under the armpit. Using
   stationary circles apply pressure
   to stretch the skin upward and
   release it downward. You're applying pressure toward the armpit, as
   that is the direction you want the
   fluid to move.

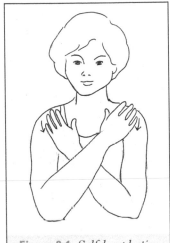

Figure 8.1. *Self-lymphatic-massage for the neck*

3. Sweep the skin from the midline (vertical watershed) of the
   chest toward the uninvolved armpit. Do this in several
   places along the chest.

4. Sweep the skin across the vertical
   watershed toward the uninvolved
   side, with each stroke moving
   down the chest from neck to
   navel. For this step you may want
   to use the pads of your fingers
   instead of the palm of your hand.

5. Sweep the skin from the involved
   armpit across the midline to the
   uninvolved armpit. Repeat
   several times across the chest
   wall. Go around scars.

6. Imagine there is a box around
   your navel (belly button). Sweep
   five times toward the navel from
   each corner of the box. Use

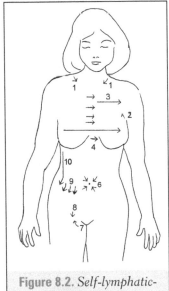

Figure 8.2. *Self-lymphatic-massage for right-arm lymphedema*

slightly firmer pressure, depressing the tissue on your belly about one inch.

7. In the groin on the *involved* side, using stationary circles, apply pressure up toward the belly button and release down.

8. On the involved side, sweep the skin from the lower horizontal watershed to the groin.

9. On the involved side, sweep the skin over the horizontal watershed.

10. On the involved side, sweep the skin from the armpit down to the groin.

Repeat step 1 as you practice abdominal breathing.

Self-Massage for Breast Swelling

If you have breast swelling, or breast and arm swelling, additional massage may help. After completing the lymph drainage to the trunk as outlined above, sweep the skin directly from the inner area of the breast toward the armpit, circling around the nipple.[6] Repeat the stroke five to ten times. You can also massage from the breast upward to the area above the collarbone, again repeating five to ten times.

Modified Trunk Massage

If you are somewhere where you can't undress but wish to stimulate your lymphatic system, you can do a mini massage of the neck area. Do five stationary circles in a couple of spots, such as on the side of the neck just under the ear and in the area above the collarbone. Then do five sweeping strokes along the top of the shoulder toward the neck. Repeat the sequence several times. This can be good to do while traveling in a car or plane. If you are at work and want to boost your lymph system, take a two-minute massage break.

Self-Massage Especially for the Arm

As mentioned before, the arm should never be massaged until *after* the neck and trunk have been massaged. Once you're ready to massage the arm, follow the steps below, which correspond to the numbers in Figures 8.3 and 8.4. Repeat each sweep five to seven times; repeat each stationary circle fifteen to twenty times.

Upper Arm

1. Sweep the skin on the outside of your arm upward, around the back of your shoulder, and into the nodes above your collarbone.

2. Sweep the skin on the inside of your upper arm upward and outward to the back of your shoulder. Sweep in three different places along the upper arm, moving down from the armpit to the elbow with each set of upward strokes (i.e., the first set of strokes is near the armpit stroking toward the outer arm and then toward the neck; the second is a little farther down; and the third set is near the elbow). Do the front of the upper arm first, then the back of the upper arm.

Elbow

3. Using stationary circles, apply pressure at the bend of your elbow to stretch the skin in an upward direction toward the shoulder; then release downward. Your stroke should be directed to the outer part of your arm.

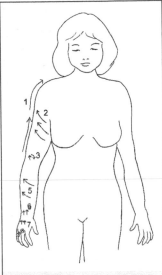

Figure 8.3. *Lymphatic massage for front of right arm*

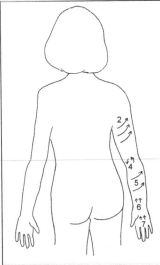

Figure 8.4. *Lymphatic massage for back of right arm*

4. If fibrosis (thickening) is present around the elbow, apply pressure a little more firmly. The tissue may soften a little during the massage. If it does, move to the next area near the elbow. If you don't notice any softening, simply move on after one minute.

Forearm

5. Sweep skin upward on the inside and outside of your forearm.

Wrist

6. Using stationary circles around the wrist, apply pressure upward and release downward, or use a sweep motion upward. Increase the pressure a little if fibrosis is present.

Hand

7. Using stationary circles, apply pressure upward and release downward on the palm and back of your hand, or use a sweep motion upward.

8. Sweep across the skin on your fingers and thumb toward the back of your hand.

Finish by raising your arm overhead. Sweep the skin from your fingertips down the back of your hand, over the wrist and forearm to the outside of your upper arm, across the back of your shoulder, and down the side of your trunk to the groin area. As with all massage, end with several abdominal breaths.

Back Massage by a Partner

Although you can do most lymphatic massage yourself, it can be helpful (and relaxing) to have someone else do it for you. This is especially true of massage to the back, where it is very awkward and not really advisable to massage yourself. Stimulating the back with lymphatic massage provides another alternative drainage pathway across the vertical watershed. The techniques and strokes follow the same guidelines as those outlined above for self-massage.

We suggest including back massage as a part of trunk massage—

that is, *before* massaging the arm. However, back massage will certainly benefit you anytime it is done, even completely by itself, without other parts of the massage. You sometimes just need to accept help when it is offered. Sit leaning over a table with pillows beneath your chest for support, arms reaching forward and forehead resting on your hands. Or lie on your stomach with your arms at your side, forehead resting on a rolled towel or small pillow.

Remind your partner to use very light, slow pressure and to always release the pressure after each stroke. Most women say their spouses use too much pressure. Perhaps it would be helpful to first perform the massage on your partner so they can feel how much pressure to use. Practice deep breathing while you are receiving the massage. Inhale through your nose and relax the abdomen as it fills with air. Exhale through pursed lips and contract the abdomen.

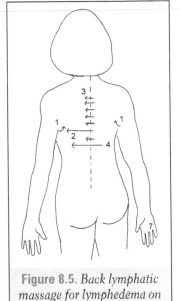

Figure 8.5. *Back lymphatic massage for lymphedema on the right side of the body*

Here is the technique, as illustrated in Figure 8.5:

1. Using stationary circles at both armpits, apply pressure upward and release downward. Do twenty repetitions.

2. Sweep the skin from the vertical watershed (midline) toward the *uninvolved* armpit in several places.

3. Sweep the skin across the vertical watershed toward the uninvolved side in several places along the spine.

4. Sweep the skin from the involved armpit across the back to the uninvolved armpit in several places.

Note from Jeannie: Self-massage is the treatment I continued (along with occasional bandaging) even after my lymphedema subsided. I still usually spend a few minutes doing it two or three times a week.

While I was learning I worked very hard to emulate the techniques Gwen used while she massaged me. I tried to duplicate the pressure she applied and to copy the types of strokes she used. I even weighed my own fingers' pressure on a postage meter—it was just six ounces. If I found an area that had become harder (fibrotic), then I dug in with a little more pressure until it softened.

I grew frustrated that I couldn't massage my own back. Then I found a solution that seemed to help. (Keep in mind, this is my idea, not something Gwen or any doctor would prescribe.) I bought a new paint roller with a super-fluffy sheath (the kind for heavily textured walls), and I learned to use it on my back. I roll from my ribs across my back and along my shoulder. Using the roller I can apply pressure in places I couldn't reach without it.

Do I feel silly using my paint roller? You bet. But it seems to help, even if the benefit is only in my mind. If you decide to try this trick, note that the lightest ones are the easiest to use, and make sure you get one that doesn't squeak!

Self-massage is an important component of managing lymphedema. It is a great idea to incorporate it into your daily routine.

9

EMMA'S STORY
PERSISTENCE PAYS OFF

Emma's voice on the other end of the phone is soft and pleasant, her speech quick. She came to the States from Mexico when she was young. She and her husband live near a large metropolitan area in the South and have four grown children. Her children don't live with her and her husband any longer, but they are still a big part of their everyday lives. When we talk about her lymphedema, frustration colors her voice. "For me, trying to find out anything about lymphedema was awful," she says. "My arm was swollen, getting bigger all the time. I was asking my doctor for help, but he didn't seem to know how to get help for me." Her doctor didn't know there was a lymphedema clinic in her area, even though she lives near a big city.

She set out to find information on her own. She searched the Internet and asked health providers. Finally her doctor came up with the name of a large facility that had a therapist treating lymphedema patients two days a week. Emma worked with the therapist for a month or so. "My arm was getting a little bit better, but not my hand. My fingers had swelled up like empanadas." She was beginning to feel hopeless. "My therapist did a little bit of work on me, then gave me a list of places to go to get compression garments. I really didn't feel like my arm was ready to be measured for garments, but I called anyway. And I found out from the person on the phone that there was a new treatment clinic not far away and she knew of some good therapists there. That's how I found Debra, my therapist now. Debra knew what to do for me."

It's been almost two months since Emma began getting MLD massage treatments. She has also learned exercises and massages she can do for herself. She bandages and wears a sleeve and a glove, and she uses a pump, paid for by insurance, every day for an hour. To concentrate on getting her lymphedema under control, she has taken a leave of absence from her job, which involves working with low-income families.

She knows she's lucky to have the time off from work, but still it has been a struggle. "With the cancer, everybody was there for me with support," she says. "But with this it's different. Nobody understands what lymphedema is and they think it's just a minor problem I will get over. I might complain to my husband"—she chuckles—"but he just doesn't understand. This is something I have to deal with and adjust to for the rest of my life. Everyone expects the same from me even though I am not the same. I have to take precautions when living everyday life so I don't make the situation worse. I am limited in what I can and cannot do, but my friends and family expect the same as before." Having lymphedema has been significant. "Sometimes I feel like getting through cancer was nothing compared to this. The cancer I could do something about and maybe feel like it was done. But this I'll have to live with my whole life."

A large percentage of the people Emma works with are Hispanic. She says, "Even though they work hard, they don't have insurance. When they get sick, a lot of the time they can get really overwhelmed and don't know what to do, but there are places, like the hospital in our city, that work with people as long as they make payments, even if they don't have insurance." Talking about a friend from Colombia who recently found a lump in her armpit, she says, "The doctors told her she had breast cancer. She told them that she didn't want chemo because she thought 'What's the use?' She was so depressed. She didn't think anybody would want her after her surgery. She didn't think she was worth having reconstruction. We talked a long time, and pretty soon I was throwing open my blouse and showing her my own reconstruction. She was in awe and asked if she could touch it. I told her yes, but that I had no feeling in it." Emma laughs. "She even remarked about the nipple, and I told her it was tattooed on but it was all mine." Her friend decided to have reconstruction and recently underwent surgery.

Emma's arm continues to improve, and so does her hand. She says, "I'm beginning to see my knuckles again." She's getting over some of her frustration, she says, "But I still have my pity days when I get down. I'm sort of worried about the night sleeve I'm getting pretty soon. I saw it. It's huge. It looks like if I turn over wrong and hit my husband with it, it's going to kill him." We both laugh.

Emma says, "A lot of Hispanic women don't want to go to the doctor, don't want to find out what's wrong with them. But you have to go. What's worse, getting sicker and dying or finding out what you can do to help yourself? You just don't want to give up. Ever."

IO

MASSAGE for SCARRING, CORDING, and MYOFASCIAL RELEASE

Launching into a discussion of scars may seem like a remote side-track from dealing with lymphedema. But scars resulting from breast cancer surgery can play a big role in limiting life after treatment. Not only can they be unsightly, but their inflexible grip can bind movement, cause pain, hinder reconstruction, and even inhibit the flow of lymph fluid. Scars are something you want to tend to. In general, treating them is a matter of stretching them, softening them, and applying pressure so they will loosen their grip. In this chapter you'll find several techniques that are literally at your fingertips for dealing with scars.

Treating scars can be easy and quite effective, particularly if your scars are fairly new. Surgeon Daniel Ladizinsky says immature scars can usually be softened using scar massage in combination with a product called CICA Care, a soft, silicone-based, adhesive gel that is applied directly to the scar. Pharmacies and drugstores sell CICA as well as many less expensive, over-the-counter scar gels. Some slightly more mature scars can be altered using myofascial release techniques, discussed later in the chapter. But for older or obstinate scars the best treatment is massage specifically designed to treat scarring.

Scar Massage

Before you begin scar massage take a few minutes to do a session of lymphatic massage. Because the purpose of scar massage is to mobilize scars and restore the normal mobility of the skin and underlying tissues, it goes deeper than lymphatic massage, and that means using a heavier pressure. Since massaging with a heavier pressure can bring on fluid, it is important to first clear the drainage pathways with lymphatic massage. After that, begin the scar massage, starting gently and gradually increasing the pressure. Although pressure is a component of breaking down scar tissue, avoid going so deeply that you cause sharp, stabbing pain. The most you should feel is a slight discomfort, a feeling of pulling, or a light burning sensation. When you're through with the scar massage, finish by again doing a few minutes of lymphatic massage.

Set aside two to three minutes a day to perform scar massage; add a little more time for the lymphatic massage before and after. You're going to want to massage all the scars on your breast, chest, and in your armpit. You may find it easier to do the massage while facing a mirror.

To begin, place the hand of the side where you had surgery on top of your head. Then place your other hand over the area where you had surgery or radiation. Slighty bend your fingers and hold them together. Use the pads of two or three fingers to perform the massage. Maintain contact with the area you are massaging. Don't let your fingers slide across the skin. For that reason, you don't want to use lotion or oil during the massage. But do apply lotion *after* the massage. Vitamin E oil is especially good for skin and for scars; you may want to apply it at night as it is quite greasy. Use a less oily lotion or cream during the day.

Start with a light pressure and then progress to a firmer stroke. You may notice one or two places that feel "stuck." Spend a little more time in those areas.

Now for the techniques:

1. Use short strokes to massage parallel to the scar on each side of it, repeating each stroke three to five times (Figure 10.1).

The pressure should be firm but not painful. Then move on to the next section of skin. Do this until you have covered the entire incision area. You can also stroke perpendicularly across the scar, from about half an inch on one side to half an inch on the other side. Repeat along the length of the scar.

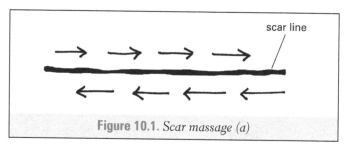

Figure 10.1. *Scar massage (a)*

2. Using one or two fingers, make circular strokes, both clockwise and counterclockwise, across the top of the scar as well as just above and below it (Figure 10.2). Repeat each stroke three to five times before moving on to the next section of skin.

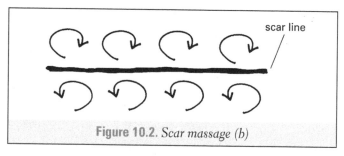

Figure 10.2. *Scar massage (b)*

Cording (Axillary Web Syndrome)

Cording, or axillary web syndrome (AWS), is a complication of axillary lymph node dissection. It is characterized by a tight and sometimes painful cord that starts in the axilla (armpit) and extends into the arm, sometimes traveling to the wrist and thumb.[1] A person with AWS can look at her armpit area in a mirror and see a web of cords underlying the skin. The area is made taut and even painful by moving the arm out to the side and raising it. The cord is thought to be composed of sclerosed (scarred or inflamed) veins and lymphatics. The phenomenon is quite common. One study reported that 6 percent of patients had developed cording in the first week following surgery. By eight weeks 95 percent of patients had developed some symptoms of the condition.[2]

Although cording is most likely to develop within eight weeks after surgery, Gwen has seen it develop much later. It can contribute to a limitation of motion in the shoulder and can be very painful. The condition doesn't seem to be related to whether or not cancer was found in the lymph nodes, but the *number* of lymph nodes removed seems to influence how extensive it becomes. In one study patients who'd had sentinel lymph node biopsy developed cording less frequently than those who'd undergone axillary lymph node dissection. For the sentinel node biopsy (SLNB) patients who developed axillary web syndrome, the symptoms did not extend as far into the arm.[1] The condition is reported to be self-limiting (meaning it will eventually resolve on its own), but that is not always the case. It can definitely benefit from therapeutic intervention. The earlier treatment is initated, the less discomfort and functional loss (loss of ability to use the arm) the patient will experience.

Treating cording involves gently stretching the axillary area. Devote a few minutes every day to working on it. Lie down with your arm raised over your head and position it so it is completely resting against a pillow. Find a position where you can feel a stretch in the affected area, but not to the point where it is painful. Use as many pillows as you need to support the arm so it can fully relax. The cording will tend to release better if your arm is supported rather than just hanging. Another idea is to take hold of an overhead kitchen cupboard or the top of a shower stall. Hang on with your fingerstips and gently rotate your body away to feel the stretch in the axilla. Again, do not cause pain. Once you're in position and can feel the stretch, practice your abdominal breathing. Imagine you are breathing oxygen into the area and breathing out the tightness and tension. Maintain the position for three or four slow breaths.

Jane M. Kepics, a physical therapist from Pennsylvania, has studied cording. Here are some of her ideas for dealing with it:[3]

* For localized pain, apply a cold pack or mild heat for no longer than ten minutes. Because you will likely have decreased sensation in the area, to protect the skin you must place pads beneath the cold pack or heat. Since heat is *not* usually good for lymphedema, do some lymphatic massage before and after applying the heat in case extra fluid builds up.

* Maintain good posture.

* Perform abdominal breathing.

* For scar-tissue release, hold your arm out slightly away from your body. With the palm of your other hand, hold onto the skin on the under side of your middle to upper arm, and simply apply traction to stretch the skin toward the elbow. Hold the stretch for at least ninety seconds, or as long as you can if your arm tires sooner.

* Do the same scar-tissue release directly over the cording in the axilla.

* Do some myofascial release (described below).

Note from Jeannie: I have cording. I can't remember when it developed but I think it may have come on not long after surgery. I believe I just didn't notice it due to my soreness and the fact that I was healing from a mastectomy. I could see the cord but I didn't think about it, even though my shoulder grew stiff and sore at times. Lately I've used the techniques described above. After only a couple weeks of working on it, the cording and stiffness seem to have gone. Gwen tells me I may need to occasionally work on it some more, as it may tighten up again before it loosens for good.

Myofascial Release

Myofascial release is another specialized massage technique that is effective in relieving symptoms of tightness, fibrosis, and cording. It has been around for a long time as a treatment for tight tissues, but only recently have we discovered how beneficial it can be after breast cancer treatment.

Myofascial release is defined as "an application of a controlled force to the soft tissue (myofascial) structures in a specific direction to stretch the tissue for the purpose of restoring or enhancing normal mobility of a restricted region."[4] Myofascial structures are the thin sheaths or layers of tissue that line muscle cells. (*Myo-* means "muscle.") You have probably seen fascia when you've handled chicken or other raw meat—it is the sticky, whitish, translucent covering that clings to the meat just beneath the skin. Tightness can develop in the myofascia following radiation treatment or surgery to the breast and axilla, even sentinel node biopsy. The scar tissue that lies under the skin covers a much larger area than the scar you can see on the surface of the skin. Myofascial release techniques can help to loosen the tightness that results from this subcutaneous (beneath the skin) scarring.

If you are working with a therapist, you can ask if she or he is familiar with myofascial release techniques. Although you can do some of this work yourself, it is easier for someone else to do it for you. Myofascial release involves using your hands to gently pull the skin *away from* the tightness. You pull only as far as the skin will allow then stay in that position, maintaining the tension for ninety seconds or longer. It might feel as though the skin is not moving very far, if at all. Even if that's the case, try to maintain a light traction on the skin while not forcing it, and do not let your fingers slide over the skin. What you are trying to do is move the top layer of skin against the layer beneath it (the myofascia). It should not be painful, but you should feel a good stretch in the tight tissues. The technique requires patience. You don't want to force it; just "be" with the stretch.

Here's how you can try the technique to deal with tightness following breast cancer treatment. Lie down and elevate your arm by resting it on a pillow over your head, or sit and rest the arm on top of your head or over the back of the couch. With your other hand find the tight areas in your chest, armpit, or ribs. First see how the skin on your *uninvolved* side moves, for a reference. Normal soft tissue should move easily in all directions. After breast cancer you will most likely find some tight tissue, even if you have full range of motion in your shoulder. You'll feel the tightness when you pull the tissue away from the scars. That is the direction in which to move your hands during myofascial stretching.

If you have cording in your armpit, place your other hand close to the armpit and just pull down and across your torso in the direction of the opposite hip. Remember, the action shouldn't hurt. Pull the tissue as far as it will move and then apply a gentle pressure against the restriction. Maintain the gentle pressure for ninety seconds. And, as if you don't have enough to do already, practice your abdominal breathing.

If you have tightness around the breast scar or mastectomy scar you can release some of it by placing your hand directly over the scar and gently stretching the skin away from it. You'll probably feel the most tightness as you stretch the skin down toward the belly.

For some patients, stretching the skin away from the scar may be too uncomfortable, or there may be areas on the skin that are still not completely healed. In that case you can try applying the pressure in the direction of the greatest ease of movement. As illogical as it may seem, maintaining a steady pressure *toward* the scar seems to loosen the myofascial tissue. Applying pressure toward the scar area is called *indirect* myofascial release technique; stretching away from the scar is called *direct* technique. Both are effective to loosen tight tissue.

Dr. Ladizinsky and Gwen recall a patient who had bilateral mastectomies (both breasts removed) for breast cancer and then received radiation to the entire chest wall. She had significant skin changes related to the surgery, and she had scar tissue from the radiation burns that developed on her chest. She was highly motivated to undergo reconstruction, but none of the tissue on her entire chest wall would move at all in any direction. Dr. Ladizinsky was doubtful there was enough mobility in the tissue to perform reconstruction, but he sent the patient to physical therapy. For two months she received myofascial release treatments. Her husband also helped daily with the techniques. After several months she had enough mobility in the tissue to allow for successful reconstruction. It was also interesting to note that she enjoyed the side benefit of having less lymphedema in her trunk and arms after the scar tissue was loosened.

Massage after Radiotherapy

Radiation therapy leaves scars of its own. It kills cancer cells, but as it does it can burn and scar the skin and the tissues beneath the skin. As radiation oncologist Jai Nautiyal explains, radiotherapy, because it penetrates the skin, can damage the lining of the small blood vessels and cause a thickening of the connective tissue (the base substance that holds everything together under the skin). To top it off radiation therapy is sneaky. Its ill effects may not appear for over a year. Gwen worked with a patient who developed scar tissue (radiation fibrosis) in the breast more than a year after completing radiation and reconstruction. The fibrosis caused a hardening, shrinking, and distortion of the reconstructed breast until its shape no longer matched that of the other breast. (In such cases massage techniques such as those described later in this chapter can help.) Because radiation fibrosis can develop so long after radiotherapy, once you've been treated it is important to continue checking your skin for hardness, thickening, or binding in the areas that have been irradiated.

For the best result from plastic surgery after breast cancer surgery and radiation, Dr. Ladizinsky says the quality of tissue is a factor. He acknowledges that scars related to surgery or radiation can be softened and stretched, resulting in tissue that can lead to better outcomes following reconstruction. Once you have completed radiotherapy, wait until the skin is well healed before beginning any massage. Then, if the tissue has become hard, tight, and bound down, you may want to begin a massage regimen to loosen it. Both scar massage and myofascial release techniques work well to stretch and soften irradiated scar tissue. The hardened areas, especially around the breast scar after a lumpectomy, need some deep-tissue work to soften them. The small circular strokes described in the section on scar massage are effective on those areas. The massage needs to be firm yet gentle. Although radiation scars seem tough, the tissue is actually fragile. Massage that is too aggressive can cause microscopic tears, which in turn can cause more scarring. Be sure to apply lotion or oil after the massage.

In a recent bit of good news, studies involving a relatively small number of patients have shown that the medication pentoxifylline has improved radiation-induced fibrosis.[5,6] You might discuss this with your physician if scarring is a problem for you.

Difficulties with reconstruction aren't the only problems radiation therapy can cause. Scarring can cause a loss of range of motion in the shoulder, even long after a patient has regained full mobility after surgery. For patients unaware of this possibility it can be quite a surprise if the shoulder becomes stiff and painful. Check the range of motion in your shoulder often—once or twice a day—for the first year after your treatment is completed.

It may seem that scars are just one more thing to deal with, but they can play a big part in your total recovery from breast cancer treatment. Tending to them can make you more comfortable, can afford greater ease of movement, and may even help lymphedema-related swelling. There's a lot that can be done about scars, and dealing with them lets us move on. And moving on is what it's all about. Read in the next chapter about how Linda moved on after working with scars that developed following her surgery.

11

LINDA'S STORY
MASSAGING SCARS and DEALING with
LYMPHEDEMA of the TORSO

On the day we first met, Linda squeezed our interview between appointments for physical therapy and lymphedema treatment. We sat in the cafeteria of the medical facility. Of medium height and build, she was dressed in jeans and a plaid, snap-button shirt that she wore untucked. At the time, Linda was in her mid-forties. Her children were still at home though they were almost grown. She had been living with her fiancé, Ron, for seven years. She spoke thoughtfully, conveying the impression that she would never utter an unplanned word. "Before I met Ron," she said, "I worked at a large corporation. I started out as an executive secretary. They promoted me to inventory and dispatching the fleet, but that didn't work out, so I quit and now I'm working with Ron managing a Kampgrounds of America (KOA) campground."

Linda's mother had had cancer eleven years before. She said, "She went through surgery, chemotherapy, and radiotherapy, but despite all that work the cancer spread to her bones." Her mother died, and two years later Linda discovered she had cancer. "I was luckier than my mother," she said with a bit of sarcasm. "They found my cancer before it had spread to my lymph nodes. I didn't have to have chemotherapy." However, just a year before we met, Linda found out she had cancer again, in the other breast. "I never felt a lump," she said. She had a mastectomy, but the surgery "didn't go well at all. Somehow they pulled a wrong tube, and a couple of days later I started to swell. I learned later the swelling was lymphedema. Then it became infected. Everything went wrong. I reacted to the antibiotics and spent four days in the hospital.

"After I was released, the infection came back. I was in the hospital for five days the second time. The swelling was terrible. And when I finally went home, I had to keep going back two or three times a week to have them aspirate the swelling. Each time, the doctor removed anywhere from a few drops of fluid to as much as a cup or two cups. That went on for six weeks. I was commuting seven or eight hundred miles a week. It was awful." The swelling did not subside; instead, it manifested in her torso. "It's still there," she told me during our first meeting. She leaned back, pulled at her shirt, and indicated a handful of flesh. "See?" She moved her hands to the other side, where there was much less bulk. "And it's down from what it used to be."

When she first got lymphedema none of her health-care practitioners seemed to know anything about it. What little information the doctor gave her only mentioned lymphedema of the arms and legs. She went to a physical therapist for problems with her jaw; the doctors thought she might have temporomandibular joint disorder (TMJ). As it turned out, she was developing a spinal problem because of the dramatic changes to her sitting and sleeping postures as a result of the swelling. The therapist thought the lymphedema was Linda's most significant problem, so she began treating her for it.

Linda's early treatment regimen included visits to the therapist one or two times a week. After a few months she started taking medication for depression, which seemed to increase her energy. She worked out on an exercise bicycle and did self-massage, including scar massage. She also used an electric massager. The idea of using it came to her on her own. She had it in her purse during our first interview. It looked like a flashlight with a rounded top about the size of a showerhead. She flipped a switch on its side and it hummed to life. She made a motion toward her waist, where she had the most swelling. "I run it between my ribs," she said. "I think it helps." Soon thereafter, between the treatments she received and her use of the massager, she was able to eliminate the bag of fluid on her belly. In an e-mail, she wrote, "The massager does all the work for me. I just have to move it around to hit all the right spots. Spending extra time directly on the hard scar tissue seems to be beneficial, too. I don't plan to feel like a sloppy, fat couch potato for much longer."

Recently, five years after our initial meeting, Linda and I spoke on the phone. She seemed more at ease than she did the first time we met. Her general health has improved. A lot of her physical problems went away when she quit working, though she still owns the campground. She struggles with lymphedema every day. "I massage, massage, massage, and I drink lots of water," she told me. "Some days my massage hits the right spot and everything moves and I feel like I've dropped fifty pounds, but other days it just doesn't work like that." She added that she's been cancer-free for eight years, the same amount of time that had passed when her cancer recurred. She said she's eager to be done with the marker symbolized by the anniversary. She's ready to leave it behind and move on.

12

COMPRESSION:
BANDAGES *and* GARMENTS

Compressing swollen tissue is another important aspect of lymphedema treatment. In this chapter we discuss the two primary methods of compression: the use of bandages and garments.

Compression Bandaging

Compression bandaging is an effective treatment for removing fluid from the area that is wrapped; as such it is a critical part of the comprehensive lymphedema treatment program. When swelling has persisted in an area, the tissue loses some of its elasticity and does not return to its original position and shape, even if the amount of fluid eventually decreases. Compression bandages apply external pressure to a swollen limb, supporting the skin and its underlying lymph vessels, and thereby helping to preserve some of the tissue's original elasticity.

It is best to work with a therapist to determine if bandaging is indicated for you, and if so, what the best type is. You shouldn't attempt bandaging on your own until you have been instructed by someone trained in the technique. What is presented here is just one example of basic bandaging. Many options and products are being developed all the time. This is another good reason to work with a lymphedema therapist who has stayed up-to-date on the latest information.

The bandages used in lymphedema treatment are rolls of short-stretch cloth that are wrapped around the involved extremity. Although they resemble sports bandages such as Ace wraps, which you are probably familiar with, they are not as stretchy. *Do not* try substituting sports bandages for them. Sports-type bandages may cause more swelling.

Bandaging normally is preceded by applying a cotton stockinette to the arm, then wrapping white gauze around the fingers, and adding a layer of soft padding to the arm. Next, different-sized short-stretch bandages are wrapped around the hand and up the arm, to within a short distance of the shoulder. The number of bandages used depends on the size of the arm and how effectively the compression is achieved, but at least three or four bandages are generally necessary.

Never wrap the bandages tight; pull just enough to take up the slack. The amount of compression is determined *not* by how tightly the bandages are wrapped but rather by how many layers of bandages are applied. The compression should be even along the whole length of the arm; if it varies (if it feels looser in one place and tighter in another) another bandage is used to even up the pressure.

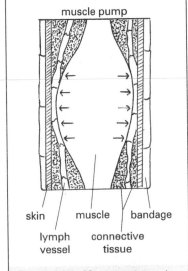

Figure 12.1. *How a compression bandage enhances a muscle's pumping action to improve lymph flow*

The Physiology of Bandaging

By using external support bandages, you can enhance other phases of treatment and ensure their success.[1] Bandaging helps by

* ✳ creating a semirigid support against which the muscle can work, improving the muscle-pumping action, and causing a contraction of the lymph vessel, all of which will move lymph fluid (Figure 12.1)[2]

* influencing the movement of fluid in the tissue channels, causing interstitial fluid to move into the functioning lymph system

* increasing total tissue pressure, which causes venous capillaries and the initial lymph vessels to take in more fluid and causes arterial capillaries to release less fluid[1]

* preventing the reaccumulation of lymph fluid in the arm

* improving and maintaining the shape of the arm (a comprehensive lymphedema treatment regimen typically causes the size of the arm to fluctuate; bandaging keeps the amount of compression consistent throughout the fluctuations, thus helping to reshape the limb)[3]

Why Can't You Use Ace Wraps, Which Are Much Less Expensive?

High-stretch elastic sports bandages, such as Ace wraps, are not effective in treating lymphedema. When the muscles are at rest, the constant compression provided by a sports bandage does not allow the lymphatic vessels to fill and thereby prevents the draining of fluid from the tissue. When the muscles contract, the sports bandage is so stretchy that it does not provide a rigid enough support for the muscles to pump against. Hence it fails to raise tissue pressure enough to effectively influence the lymphatic pump.[2]

Guidelines for Compression Bandaging

Here are some guidelines that can help to ensure success in bandaging:

* Fingers should be wrapped separately in gauze bandages about one to two inches wide (Figure 12.2).[3] The gauze used is a special type made for this purpose that can be obtained from any supplier of lymphedema bandages. Special small cloth bandages are also available for this purpose; they last longer than gauze and are easier to wash.

✳ Greater pressure should be applied to the hand and lower forearm, with a gradual reduction in pressure as you move up the limb toward the trunk. Remember, greater pressure is achieved *not* by applying bandages more tightly at the hand and forearm but rather by applying more layers and more overlap of bandages in those areas (Figure 12.3).[2]

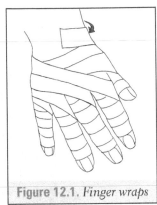

Figure 12.1. *Finger wraps*

✳ The width of the bandages used varies depending on the circumference of the arm. (Bandages come in widths of four, six, eight, ten, and twelve centimeters; five centimeters approximately equals two inches.) The number of bandages used varies with the size and shape of the arm and the person's tolerance.

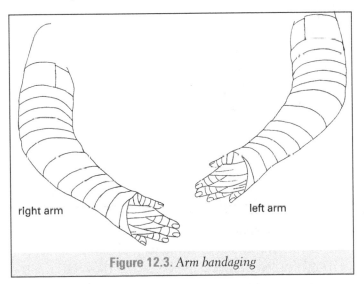

right arm　　　　　　　　　　　　　left arm

Figure 12.3. *Arm bandaging*

✳ Applying appropriate padding beneath the bandages is necessary to protect the skin and bony prominences, and to provide an even distribution of pressure over the entire limb. Padding also prevents chafing and protects tender areas. Your therapist may use any of several good padding materials that are available; one is a soft cotton padding called Artiflex.

* Foam padding may be applied to shape the limb, or denser foam used to break down fibrotic areas. Foam of different densities can be cut into small pieces and placed in a small "chip" bag, which can be placed over areas of fibrosis or hardening. (Dr. Vodder's School calls the chips "chocolates.") There are unlimited ways to use pieces of foam, so don't be surprised by your therapist's creativity. Premade foam pads or chip bags are also available—for example Jovi Paks and Swell Spots, which come in all shapes and sizes.

* Soft compression sleeves are available that look like giant oven mitts and have foam built in to promote fluid drainage. You can bandage over the sleeve, or it may come with a nylon outer sleeve that maintains the compression. These devices are quite bulky, so many patients wear them only at night. Some people find them much easier to use than bandages and thus may comply more readily with their use. Several of the suppliers of lymphedema products listed in Resources offer a sleeve of this type. Examples include the Tribute sleeve, Jovi Pak, or OptiFlow. CircAid also offers a similar product.

* If there is swelling in the trunk, bandaging there can be helpful. The January–March 2004 newsletter of the National Lymphedema Network suggests using two rolls of medium-stretch bandages rather than the short-stretch bandages that are used on the arm. Bandages with higher elasticity are needed to facilitate fluid movement since the trunk has less muscle-pumping action than the arm. It may also be useful to apply foam pads or strips to help move fluid across the watershed.[4] A sports bra or other lymphedema bra may be used either by itself to provide extra compression against the trunk or over the bandages to hold them in place.

When Should You Bandage?

When you bandage will likely vary depending on your therapist's preferences, where the therapist received training, how much treatment you have already received, how your arm is responding, and whether you are also using a support garment (discussed later). Again, you should not try to bandage yourself until you have been instructed by a therapist specially trained in bandaging and lymphatic massage. If done improperly, bandaging can cause fluid buildup in the wrong areas or can cause constriction, blocking the flow of fluid.

Most therapists will recommend that you wear bandages twenty-four hours a day during the intensive phase of therapy, taking them off only to bathe and to receive treatment.[5,6,7] Once you are in the maintenance phase and wearing a support garment, you may be able to gradually discontinue regular use of bandages. Other therapists suggest wearing bandages while you sleep for several months after you have completed an intensive course of treatment. Some suggest using them if you are exercising or performing physical activity. Some suggest wearing them after you have had lymphatic massage.[8]

After successfully completing lymphedema treatment, some patients only use bandages while exercising or to deal with episodes of swelling. Bandaging for a few days can be effective if you notice symptoms of increased fluid in the area, such as heaviness, pressure, fullness, achiness, numbness, or tingling. When the symptoms have decreased, the bandaging can be discontinued. Many wear bandages when they may be at higher risk for swelling, such as during the summer or when they are traveling by air (see Chapter 5, "Preventing Lymphedema").

Some patients believe that since elevating the arm helps with swelling, it is safe to remove their bandages and/or garments when they sleep. In fact, wearing bandages can be most helpful then, since during sleep the muscles' action decreases, diminishing their pumping influence to the lymph vessels, an effect that can cause the fluid to pool rather than to move through the lymph system.[9]

It is probably a good idea to experiment. See what works best for you and is realistic for your lifestyle. Certainly, the more you wear bandages, the better the results will be. However, we know that many people simply cannot or will not wear bandages twenty-four hours a day. They can still achieve some benefit from bandaging. Many patients are happy to see even small or moderate reductions in swelling and find this result satisfactory. Others are satisfied simply knowing they have the option of doing more to decrease the swelling, even if they choose not to. Everyone has her own attitude about the results she can live with.

However long and however often you wear them, bandages will offer some benefit—and that is better than if you never wore them at all.

When Should You Not Bandage?

There are times when bandaging is not recommended, even if you are experiencing swelling. Some of them are listed below:

* *If you have an active infection in the area affected by lymphedema.* In the case of infection you should temporarily discontinue bandaging until the infection is under control. If you have any open wound it is important to first have it properly dressed and then to apply short-stretch bandages over the dressing. Lymphatic bandaging will actually help with wound healing, but it should be done only under medical supervision.

* *If you have circulatory problems, nerve problems, or problems with arterial insufficiency.*

* *If you feel pain.* Although the bandages are not likely to be the most comfortable things you have ever worn, they should not cause any significant pain or numbness. If they do, discontinue their use until you can discuss the issue with your therapist or doctor. Before removing the bandages, however, try going through the simple lymph-drainage exercises outlined in Chapter 16 to see if the pain or numbness diminishes with movement.

✳ *If you have a DVT (blood clot) in your arm.* Blood clots are much more common in the leg, but they can occur in the arm. They need to be considered as a possible cause whenever there is a rapid, painful onset of swelling in the arm, especially after a period of inactivity. When a clot occurs, anticoagulant medication is prescribed and will be continued for a long time, perhaps indefinitely. The usual recommendation is to wait until the clot is clearly resolving and you have been on medication for several weeks before considering resuming bandaging or lymphatic massage. Your physician should definitely be consulted about when it is safe to resume these therapies.

In the past it was recommended that women with active cancer should discontinue bandaging, but this is no longer the case. Most lymphedema experts currently believe that bandaging will not move cancer cells to other areas. There may be some circumstances in which bandaging needs to be put on hold, such as when treating the cancer is the priority, but treatment for lymphedema can be resumed as soon as it can be tolerated. If there is any question about using bandages, it is advisable to discuss the matter with your doctor and therapist.

Care of Bandages

To clean the bandages we suggest putting them in the type of net laundry bags used for socks or underclothing and washing them with a mild detergent on the gentle cycle in lukewarm water. They can be dried in the dryer on the gentle cycle; however, they will last longer if they are laid out flat and air-dried. Launder them at least every three or four days, or more frequently if they become soiled or soaked with perspiration.

Note from Jeannie: Because lymphedema was so frightening to me, I found it difficult to resume my normal life. Everything seemed to pose the possibility of making it worse. But slowly my confidence returned as I experimented with adding activities—sometimes holding my breath while doing so—and observed the effects they had on my swelling. Though I no longer need to bandage every day, as I did at the start of treatment, I still wrap when I'm going to be doing something strenuous like cleaning the house or gardening. I have a set of bandages that is stained green from the day I put in geraniums and is splattered off-white from when I painted the kitchen. So far— knock on wood—hard work doesn't seem to hurt me. In fact, if I bandage, my arm seems to benefit from a day of heavy effort. By now, I don't think there's any activity I can't do because of swelling, but I do take the precautions Gwen describes throughout the book.

Compression Garments

Since the elasticity of the skin is damaged by lymphedema, it is hard to maintain a reduction in swelling without applying some additional support to the arm. The goal at this stage is to apply sufficient compression to prevent fluid from reaccumulating after the swelling has been reduced by bandages and other components of treatment. In the first, intensive phases of treatment compression is normally achieved through the use of bandages. After the affected extremity has decreased in size, most patients should be fitted with a compression garment (sleeve and glove or gauntlet), to be worn during the daytime (although some therapists recommend wearing the garment at night as well).Compression garments are less bulky than bandages and are usually more comfortable. Standard versions are designed not to reduce swelling but to maintain the size of the limb and to prevent swelling from increasing or returning.[10] (However, some garments are now available that can help to reduce swelling.) For optimal ongoing lymphedema management, consistent and long-term use of compression garments is encouraged.[11]

Finding the Right Garment for You

There are several things to consider when selecting a garment, including your age, independence level, dexterity, lifestyle, and even environmental factors such as climate.[12] A garment is only beneficial if the patient is able to put it on and use it. Ready-to-wear garments, if you can find one to fit your arm, are less expensive and most likely will be available right away. However, sometimes it is not possible to get a good fit with a ready-made garment. In that case you'll need a custom-made garment. They are generally more expensive and take a couple of weeks to obtain after ordering, but they may be the best choice for you. Another advantage of custom-made garments is that they can be constructed with modifications that will ensure a better fit, such as extra fabric at the elbow crease or a silicone band around the top.

Garments come in different styles; the one you should get depends on the distribution of the swelling, among other things. One style fits from the wrist to the armpit; another fits from the wrist to the top of the shoulder and is secured in place with a body strap. Most people also need a garment for the hand. These, too, come in different styles. One covers just the palm, the back of the hand, and

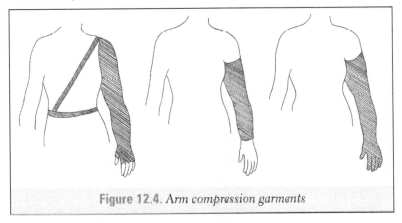

Figure 12.4. *Arm compression garments*

part of the thumb, leaving the fingers fully exposed. Another covers the palm, the back of the hand, and the bottom part of all the fingers. A third type is like a full glove. Hand garments can be either attached to the sleeve or worn separately. (See Figure 12.4.)

If you have trouble with the sleeve slipping down your arm, you might want to consider a garment with a silicone band or silicone beads at the top, which are designed to cling to the skin to hold the garment up. However, in some women the silicone band can cause a tourniquet effect. Another helpful option for holding the garment in place may be body glue, which can be obtained through medical supply companies that sell garments. Garments that include a body strap stay in place well, but this style isn't used very frequently because the part of the garment that goes over the shoulder provides no compression, and some women complain about the body straps being awkward. Again, what will work best depends on the distribution of the swelling. It is also important to pay attention to how your arm responds to the style you choose. Remember that the garment is an essential component of treatment, so it must fit correctly.

You have choices about the type of fabric a garment is made from. Garments come in versions for sensitive skin, in lighter weights for use in warm weather, in varying levels of durability, and in different colors. They may or may not have seams. Seamless garments, if available, are usually preferred because most patients find them more comfortable and thus easier to wear.

Garments differ in how much compression they provide. The most common pressure used in an arm garment is 30–40 mm Hg. (Leg garments may need to have a higher pressure.) A lighter pressure, such as 20–30 mm Hg, may be used if the patient has only mild swelling or plans to wear the garment for prevention during flying or exercising. And some individuals simply don't tolerate garments with higher levels of pressure.[12] If your lymphedema is severe you may require a garment with a pressure as high as 40–50 mm Hg. A garment called the Elvarex, made by BSN-Jobst, has a heavier weave and tends to provide more compression. Many patients find that it affords a better fit, feels more comfortable, and lasts longer than standard, lower-compression garments. Juzo has recently developed the Juzo Strong, which also provides more compression. Higher-compression garments tend to be more expensive, but, as mentioned at the beginning of this section, they have the added benefit of being able to help reduce swelling to some degree.

Several U.S. manufacturers make compression garments, and they are often available at medical supply retailers. But, again, to get the right fit, be sure to work with someone who is familiar with compression garments, ideally a certified fitter. In many cases your lymphedema therapist will be able to measure you or guide you about where to go to get measured. There is a list of manufacturers and distributors of compression garments in the Resources section at the back of the book.

Guidelines for Wearing Garments

Generally speaking, compression garments are worn under the clothing from the time you wake up until bedtime. (If you are bandaging at night, you will remove your garment in the early evening and apply bandages to wear until morning.) In the past, few therapists have recommended wearing garments at night, but that is changing.

Garments should be replaced when they are too tight, are too loose, are baggy due to age, or have otherwise lost the ability to prevent the limb from refilling. Many patients who still bandage at night can expect ongoing gradual reductions in limb size such that within two months they may need to change the size of garment they wear. With light wear and tear, garments may last as long as six months, but they often need to be replaced sooner than that.

It is suggested that you have two garments at any given time and alternate their use on a daily basis. You can wash one while wearing the other. We suggest waiting to order a second garment until you are certain the first one fits well.

The garment should feel firm and supportive, *not painful*. It should not cause the fingers to turn a dusky purple or blue. If you experience aching in your arm after a period of inactivity, rather than removing the sleeve try moving around and exercising the limb. The discomfort may be caused by a buildup of fluid and may decrease once you are active. If a tight band of constriction develops when you wear the garment, it may be a sign of a poorly fitting garment. A garment that does not fit well can actually contribute to more swelling and can be harmful to the arm.[13] Consult your therapist if any such problems arise.

Applying and Removing the Garment

Although you will most likely feel awkward the first few times you put on a garment, with practice it does get easier. Here are some suggestions that should help:

* Apply and remove the garment carefully to preserve its elasticity.

* Put on the garment when you first get up in the morning. If you wait until later in the morning your arm may have swollen and the garment may not fit properly. Avoid putting it on immediately after a bath; the moist skin and slightly increased swelling will make doing so a struggle.

* Before you put on the garment dry-lubricate your skin by dusting it with talcum powder.

* Turn the sleeve of the garment partly inside out. Pull on the folded garment until the bottom of it is past the wrist, and then unroll the top half over the elbow and upper arm.

* Get a good grip on the fabric of the sleeve by wearing a rubber glove to inch it up the arm bit by bit. Using rubber gloves can also help prevent expensive runs in the garment.

* Put a slippery plastic sleeve on your lower arm to help the garment slide over the skin. Once the garment is on, pull the plastic out from underneath it. Plastic sleeves will most likely be available where you purchase the garment.

* Once you have the folded garment above the wrist, place your hand flat against the wall at shoulder level and lean into it as you pull the garment up.

Once the garment is on, follow these general guidelines:

* Make sure the garment is smooth, without wrinkles or folds, and the fabric is distributed evenly across the limb. Wrinkles can irritate the skin or, worse, can act like elastic bands and cause fluid buildup.[13] You can use the rubber glove to help smooth out wrinkles or to pull the fabric away from the elbow crease.

* Check the garment throughout the day and pull up the sleeve if it has slid down. If necessary use skin adhesive to help the garment stay up. If you use skin adhesive, apply it

in vertical strips in several spots on the arm. Applying it horizontally can create a tourniquet effect.

* Remove the garment by taking hold of the top and pulling it down over the limb so that it ends up inside out. Be sure to inspect your skin after removing the garment. Look for any areas of redness, irritation, or dryness.

* Avoid using lotion under the garment unless it is a medical ointment or unless the garment manufacturer specifically says you can use salves, lotions, or oils. A silicone-based lotion is available that is specifically designed for use under garments. It keeps moisture in yet doesn't damage the garment. To find this product check with the garment manufacturer. Use moisturizing lotions at night, when you're not wearing the garment.

Garment Care

A clean garment will last longer. Skin oils and dirt buildup will break down the resilience of its fibers. Wearing gloves or protective clothing over the garment when performing some indoor and outdoor activities may help to keep it clean.

You can wash the garment by hand or machine. If you machine-wash it, use a gentle cycle and a mild soap. A soap made specifically for compression garments, called Variance, advertises that it gives garments a longer life. It is frequently available where compression garments are sold, or you can order it from some of the suppliers listed in the Resources section. Do not use Woolite, bleach, or fabric softeners. Launder the garment as you would any fine lingerie. Rinse it well, and roll or pat it dry in a towel. Do not twist it. Some brands of garments can be dried by machine using wash-and-wear settings. Other manufacturers suggest air-drying them.

Specialty Garments

New options are available for patients who have trouble with bandaging or who desire additional help in maintaining a reduction in swelling after lymphedema treatment. Several garments now on the market are constructed with a padded underlayer and a top layer of overlapping flaps that are tightened with Velcro cinches. These specialty garments are easier and faster to apply, have adjustable pressure, and are more comfortable for some people. These are usually worn only at night. At the same time, they are very expensive, bulkier than conventional garments, and may not be paid for by insurance. Examples include the Arm Assist, the Reid Sleeve, and the CircAid (see Resources). You can talk with your therapist to determine if a specialty garment is an option for you.

The Resources, located at the back of the book, lists suppliers of garments, bandages, and other products designed to help lymphedema. In addition, compression garments are now available over the Internet. However, we have no personal experience with this method of finding them, and we recommend caution. Let us emphasize again how important it is to get measured by a professional before purchasing a compression garment from any source. It is very difficult to measure and apply a garment by yourself, especially if you have never worn one before. A poorly fitting garment can worsen lymphedema. Once you have had one garment, you will have some idea of what works for you and what you would like in a future garment; at that point purchasing one over the Internet may be a good choice.

13

KINESIO TAPING and PUMPS

There are other treatments available that can be complimentary to standard lymphedema treatment. Kinesio Taping and vasopneumatic pumps are both effective techniques that can provide additional treatment benefits for many patients. It should be noted, though, that they should be utilized as adjuncts to a comprehensive treatment program and not as a single treatment modality.

Kinesio Taping

The past few years have seen the development of several new technologies in the treatment of lymphedema, one of which is the Kinesio Taping Method. Kinesio Taping seems to be especially effective when used in conjunction with standard CDT (complete decongestive therapy; see Chapter 6). When properly applied, the highly elastic Kinesio Tex Tape mobilizes and massages the skin to move fluid and stimulate the lymphatic system, in much the same way lymphatic massage (MLD) does. For this reason Kinesio Taping is becoming an accepted treatment for many conditions, including lymphedema. As mentioned, however, it does not replace any of the components of lymphedema therapy, but is only a supplement to it. And, like any therapy, it has to be put to use to work.

Kinesio Tex Tape and the Kinesio Taping Method (also called Kinesio Taping) were developed many years ago by Dr. Kenzo Kase, a chiropractor in Japan.[1] Kinesio Taping was already being used for a multitude of health issues in Japan when it was discovered by Olympic volleyball players in the mid-1990s. It quickly spread to use in other sports. In fact, you may have noticed many athletes, particularly gymnasts and swimmers, using the tape during the Athens Olympics. As opposed to the types of tape that are traditionally used by athletes, which are stiff and immobilize tissue, Kinesiotape is flexible and designed to move as you move. According to a book by Dr. Kase, "Kinesio Taping is based on a philosophy that aims to give free range of motion in order to allow the body's system to heal itself bio-mechanically."[2]

Ruth Coopee, who is an occupational therapist, a certified Vodder MLD/CDT therapist, a hand therapist, and a Kinesio Taping instructor, has pioneered the use of Kinesio Taping for lymphedema. She says, "When applied properly, Kinesiotape can reduce pain and has a neurological and physical affect on lymph, muscle, skin, and fascia." (As we described in Chapter 10, the fascia is the thin layer of tissue that lies just under the skin and lines the muscle.)

The Physiology of Kinesio Taping

Remember from Chapter 3, on lymphatic anatomy, that the microscopic lymph capillaries have flaps that open and close to help move the lymph fluid along. The capillaries rely on skin movement, specifically the stretching of skin, to accomplish this function. Kinesio Taping enhances the movement of skin, which in turn improves the capillaries' performance in aiding lymph flow.

Ruth Coopee outlines how Kinesio Taping stimulates lymphatic function:

* The elastic property of the tape lifts the skin and creates a gentle massage.

* Changes in interstitial pressure, combined with skin movement, open and close the initial lymphatic vessels via filaments attached to the skin.

* Taping also affects the muscle, thereby enhancing the deeper lymphatic mechanism, i.e., the "muscle pump."

* The subsequent reduction in edema (fluid buildup) removes heat and chemical substances from the tissues, improving circulation and reducing trigger points (painful spots).

* The decreased pressure on chemical receptors reduces pain and improves the return of normal sensation.

General Guidelines for Using Kinesiotape

Gwen remembers when she first encountered someone wearing Kinesiotape many years ago. She was on a small ship in the Alaskan Inland Passage on a kayaking tour and noticed a passenger with a compression sleeve. They became acquainted, and after Gwen mentioned her occupation the two launched into a long, friendly discussion about lymphedema. Gwen noticed some blue-colored strips above the neckline of the woman's blouse (Kinesio Tex Tape comes in hot pink, blue, and beige). The woman described it as her lymphedema tape. In just a few moments Gwen was peeking inside her shipmate's shirt, and the woman was happily undressing, explaining about the tape and how it worked. As soon as Gwen got home she researched the "lymphedema tape." Later, she attended one of Ruth Coopee's training courses and has used Kinesiotape extensively since then.

Many patients have successfully reduced swelling with regular use of Kinesio Taping. It seems most effective when it is applied to the places on the body where applying compression bandages or garments is difficult due to inaccessibility, such as on the trunk or breast or over the top of the shoulder. It is also useful when applied to the fingers or toes when the use of compression gloves or bandages is poorly tolerated. One application of tape will last for three to five days and can be worn in the shower. Because it is made of a cotton fabric that absorbs liquid, bath soaps, and shampoos, be sure to rinse thoroughly to avoid "soap itch," and pat dry instead of wiping to avoid lifting the edges of the tape. When spreading hand lotions, oil, or soaps, try to avoid the tape as these products can loosen the adhesive.

Remove the tape with care because it adheres to the superficial layers of skin and if pulled upward may rupture the small capillary bed underneath. As best you can, try to hold down the skin as you brush-roll the tape off. Brush-roll in the direction in which your hair grows.

Though you can wear the tape in comfort for several days, and can easily sleep, dress, and shower or bathe while wearing it, it has some limitations. Putting it on may be inconvenient, and people in public may notice that you're wearing it. But, of course, if the tape sits unused in a drawer, you're not getting any help from it at all.

Gwen has a story about the being-seen-in-public issue. As part of a class she attended, students applied Kinesio Tape to each other. Afterward, to see how it felt to wear the tape for a few days, Gwen left a patch of flesh-colored tape on her neck, a length of pink tape on her arm, and a piece of blue tape on her leg. While she was at the airport on her way home, she got some questioning stares but didn't worry about it. One young woman, who was covered with tattoos and body piercings, noticed the tape and, after a couple of minutes, leaned over and said, "That tape is really cool. Where can I get some?"

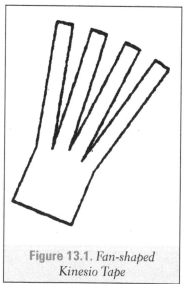

Figure 13.1. *Fan-shaped Kinesio Tape*

Taping Techniques

According to Ruth Coopee, "Typically the tape is anchored in one location and applied with 25 percent tension to stretched skin." In one technique the tape is cut in a fan shape to spread across a large area of skin (Figure 13.1). When the wearer moves, the recoiling action of the tape lifts and mobilizes the skin to stimulate lymph flow, as described above. Applied to areas of fibrosis, the fan-shaped configuration can also improve tissue mobility and soften the dense, concentrated lymph.

An especially effective technique is to cut the tape in a fan shape and apply it across the trunk from a swollen breast to the other side of the chest, or upward to the area just above the collarbone. One patient came in with a markedly swollen breast months after radiation. In a single therapy session, the taping brought her significant relief; she was unaware of just how much until she removed it three days later and could feel the fluid returning to the breast. Another technique is to use the fan-shaped tape to

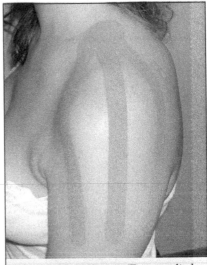

Figure 13.2. *Kinesio Tape applied over the shoulder*

treat a "pouch" of fluid that has accumulated under the armpit. Applied correctly, the tape pulls fluid from the pouch across the middle of the back to the side that has functioning lymphatics.

Kinesio Taping can also be effective when worn on the upper arm where the compression sleeve ends. The tape is applied from the upper arm to just above the collarbone (Figure 13.2). This application worked well for a patient whose job at a post office involved using her arms extensively. She wore a compression garment on her arm but still had swelling. After she added tape over the top of her shoulder, she noticed a significant decrease in swelling. In fact, some of the time she was able to manage her swelling without wearing the sleeve, as long as she was careful to pace herself and modify some of her activities. She said it was especially nice in the summer to be able to go without the sleeve and wear only the tape. This same patient later endured a breast abscess and subsequent swelling that lasted for many weeks. After the infection was resolved, she used tape on her breast and successfully drained off the extra fluid.

A special taping technique can reduce the swelling of hand edema. Cut a length of tape long enough to cover the arm from

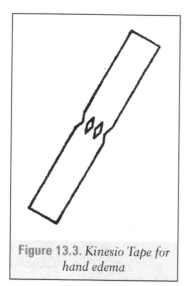

Figure 13.3. *Kinesio Tape for hand edema*

elbow to knuckle, then fold it in half crosswise. At the fold, cut two triangular holes large enough to put your fingers through (Figure 13.3). Place your fingers through the holes and apply the tape to your palm and the back of your hand.

Gwen worked with a dentist who developed swelling in her hand and fingers after a paper cut, two years following her breast cancer treatment. The woman's doctor referred her to physical therapy for lymphedema treatment. She gained some benefit from massage, exercise, and bandaging, but still had some persistent swelling. She was worried that the lymphedema would jeopardize her work, as it would have been very awkward to wear a compression glove while practicing dentistry. Gwen applied Kinesiotape to the woman's hand, and within twenty-four hours the swelling in her hand and fingers reduced more than it had following the other treatments. After a few weeks of combining all the therapies, her hand returned to normal. She still keeps tape around in case she has a flare-up. She feels her results with taping were impressive and cheerfully reports, "Kinesiotape worked for me!"

When Should You Not Use Kinesiotape?

According to Ruth Coopee, Kinesio Taping should be avoided under the following circumstances:

- ✳ If, following radiation, you have tissue that is fragile or healing and/or sensitive skin

- ✳ If you have cellulitis or infection

- ✳ In case of malignancy (active cancer)

- ✳ In case of active tuberculosis

- ✳ On open wounds

Some people may be sensitive to the tape. To make sure you're not, test a small patch of tape on an area of the body that has no lymphedema, and wait a day to see if there's a reaction. Gwen has seen a couple of people experience blistering within twenty-four hours of applying the tape. It may seem obvious, but tape should not be used if you are sensitive to it. Besides blistering, watch for the following signs of sensitivity:

* A burning sensation

* Itching

* Redness

* Discomfort

If you experience any suspicious or adverse reaction, remove the tape immediately. Remember to brush-roll it off your skin gently and slowly.

Kinesio Tex Tape can be purchased directly from some of the suppliers listed in the Resources section; however, before buying any we *strongly* recommend that you see a therapist who is trained in the Kinesio Taping Method. To be effective, the tape needs to be applied properly, and it is important to make sure you have no skin reaction to it. When a therapist is first applying the tape there may be some trial and error to determine which techniques and locations are most beneficial for you. Work with your therapist, learn how to use the tape, let your therapist test it on you, get proper instruction—then you can purchase tape on your own in the future.

The Kinesio Taping Method is another tool in the overall treatment of lymphedema. We owe thanks to Dr. Kase for developing the technique and to Ruth Coopee for sharing her knowledge of it with the community of therapists and patients working and living with lymphedema.

Vasopneumatic Pumps

Though they are now used less frequently, vasopneumatic pumps have been used for over twenty-five years in the treatment of lymphedema. In fact, up until the 1990s or so, pumps and compression garments were the only treatments available. Though other, more effective treatments have emerged, pumps are still being prescribed by some doctors and used by many people with lymphedema.

The pump is an electric, pneumatic compression device. It consists of a small air pump attached by plastic tubing to an inflatable sleeve that fits over the arm or leg. The motor forces air into the sleeve, causing it to inflate; after a specified number of seconds the motor turns off, allowing the sleeve to deflate. The cycle of inflation and deflation continues as long as the machine is on. The pump is programmed to inflate the sleeve starting at the most distal (farthest) part from the shoulder—that is, at the fingers—and to subsequently inflate each section of the sleeve, moving up the arm toward the shoulder. The goal is to "milk" the lymph fluid out of the swollen extremity.

Pumps are rarely used anymore as the sole treatment for lymphedema. Dr. Michael Foeldi, world-renowned in the field of lymphology, says that to squeeze fluid from an extremity with lymphedema toward an area that has been subjected to regional lymph node dissection "defies an understanding of basic anatomy and physiology."[3] The lymphatic system is arranged so that lymph fluid from both the arm and trunk that are located on one side of the body flows into the same set of axillary (underarm) nodes, which may have been removed during surgery or damaged by radiotherapy. The pump's action of pushing fluid from the arm into the trunk simply increases the swelling in the trunk or shoulder on that side. The pump does nothing to move the protein-rich lymph fluid into a different lymphatic quadrant that could drain the fluid away or break down the impurities.[4] Think of a swimming pool that has no drain. If you pump water from the deep end to the shallow end, it will eventually filter back to the deep end. To decrease the volume of water in the pool, the pump needs to drain *outside* the pool. It is the same with lymphedema. Without drainage, the fluid often quickly filters back to the arm when the person stops using the compression pump.

Recent improvements may have improved the effectiveness of pneumatic pumps. The sleeves of most older versions covered only the arm or the leg, but some of the newer devices now extend onto the trunk, where they pretreat and stimulate the lymphatics located there. Only after the pretreatment is complete do they begin pumping fluid from the distal area (fingers and hand) toward the shoulder. In this way the action of the newer designs more closely matches the manual lymph drainage sequence. The Flexitouch, which has recently come on the market, affords a mechanized rolling-massage action, again based on MLD principles.

Precautions when Using the Pump

Presenters and attendees at the 1993 International Congress of Lymphology generally agreed that a pump used alone is an ineffective treatment for lymphedema. If a pump is used at all, it should be used in conjunction with MLD and a comprehensive treatment program and should be set at a low pressure.[5] A study done at Stanford in 2002 showed that intermittent pneumatic compression combined with decongestive lymphatic therapy provided significantly more positive results than decongestive lymphatic therapy alone.[6]

Ongoing use of a compression pump without doing lymphatic massage, however, can pose problems, particularly in the development of fibrosis (thickening) when the fluid accumulates and concentrates at the top of the arm. The 1995 Consensus Document of the International Society of Lymphology suggests that care must be taken to prevent the patient from developing a fibrosclerotic ring around the arm where the inflatable sleeve ends.[7]

Additionally, the pump may damage remaining, healthy lymph vessels if used at higher pressures.[8] If a pump is ineffective in reducing swelling, or if swelling returns immediately, patients commonly increase the pressure in the pump or increase the time spent using it. The increased pressures are often too great for the fragile lymphatic vessels and can damage them. At a minimum, higher pressure compresses the vessels, preventing them from working.

Patients frequently report that home use of the pump works for a while and then gradually becomes less and less effective as fibrosis develops or lymphatic pathways become damaged. As it becomes less effective, they get discouraged and eventually discontinue its use. Any therapist who works a great deal with lymphedema will know of a patient who has an old pump in the closet or for sale.

Again, we would discourage people from using a pump without lymphatic massage and the other components of a complete decongestive therapy program. If you do use a pump, please consider the following guidelines:

* Use a pump *only* under the supervision of a therapist trained in comprehensive lymphatic treatment.

* Use a pump with segmental gradient compression that starts at the fingers and moves up toward the shoulder. A pump that stimulates the trunk before beginning compression in the arm is preferable.

* Use the pump in combination with a comprehensive treatment program that includes lymphatic drainage, bandaging, and exercise.

* Keep the pressure low—never higher than 35 mm Hg.

* Practice self-massage to the neck and trunk before, during, and after pumping. It is very important to clear an area for the fluid to move into. It is recommended that patients massage the trunk and top of the shoulder every five to ten minutes during pumping.[9]

* Never use a pump if you have swelling in the trunk.

* Especially with primary lymphedema, be cautious; watch closely for problems. It is best to use the pump during the first session for no longer than twenty to thirty minutes and then, if no problems develop, to slowly increase the time by ten minutes per session until you're at one hour.[9]

* Never use the pump if you have an infection anywhere in the body.

* Discontinue use of the pump if it causes pain

* If your physician recommends a compression pump without recommending any other treatments, ask about other

options. Share with your doctor any information you have regarding complex decongestive therapy. Contact the National Lymphedema Network or check the Internet to obtain information that might further educate your physician.

Distributors for pumps are listed in the Resources section. If you choose to use one, make sure you are well educated in the best way to do so.

In the next chapter Nancy details her experiences with several different types of compression. After that Carolyn recounts her experience using a pump.

14

NANCY'S STORY
a NURSE USES COMPRESSION to TREAT
HER LYMPHEDEMA

Nancy is a nurse in radiation oncology. When we first met five years ago, she wedged our interview, which took place at the clinic where she worked, into her busy Friday-afternoon schedule. She was forty at the time, but her countenance had the freshness of an undergraduate's. Her light-blue eyes sparkled brightly, her skin was clear, her cheeks were a high-colored rose. She wore a nurse's sensible shoes and a blue tunic with drawstring slacks. Over the tunic she wore a sweater.

Her cancer diagnosis had come four years before. She said, "I knew right from the start that I had cancer. I found a lump and just knew it right away." She went in for a mammogram. "The cancer didn't show up, but the lymph nodes were bright as neon." She spoke clearly and dispassionately, as if this were something that had happened to a patient of hers. "There was no history of breast cancer in my family, so it was not something that had been on my mind."

Nancy was diagnosed with stage II cancer. The surgeon aspirated both the tumor and the lymph nodes because the nodes were palpable. Eleven nodes were removed, and all tested positive, so her prognosis was poor. She participated in a clinical trial for high-dose chemotherapy and donated her own bone marrow for later transplant. Her treatments started with four months of chemotherapy followed by high-dose chemotherapy. She was in the hospital for twenty-one days. Seven months later she began treatments with radiation. "Because of my prognosis, four fields—pretty much the maximum—were radiated." She had been working in intensive care, but shortly after her cancer treatments ended she accepted a position in radiation oncology. She told me, "I feel I can tell patients who come in, 'I've been there, I can help you through this.' I see the calming effect that has."

She continued, "I was always one of the healthiest people I knew. Until I got breast cancer, I'd never had health problems. Then it seemed like everything happened. A year after I was done with the cancer treatments, I got carpal tunnel. It was in my right wrist, the same side as my breast cancer. I was lucky, I guess, because I didn't have lymphedema at the time, though I told the surgeon lymphedema might be a problem and he took some precautions."

She and her husband went for a short vacation in the country. The woman who ran the bed and breakfast where they stayed had lymphedema. "Every evening we'd see her in the family room of the house with her arm elevated on pillows and encased in a pump," Nancy said. "She'd gone to a conference at Stanford and she knew tons about lymphedema. I learned a lot from her. She attributed her lymphedema to a flu shot she'd had in that arm—she said she just didn't think about it. After hearing her story, I was much more aware of the seriousness of lymphedema. Because I'd been in a different field throughout my nursing career up to that point, I'd never really seen women who had it."

Nancy's own lymphedema came on nearly two years after she finished cancer treatments. As we talked she slipped her sweater off and showed me both arms. Though there was no swelling in her hand, one arm was somewhat larger than the other. Once lymphedema set in, she grew frustrated and scared that it would get out of control. "I was lucky I was in medicine," she said, "and lucky because I met that woman on my trip. I had some idea of what to do."

She began to elevate her arm as much as possible. She received lymphatic massage every other day for two or three weeks but didn't see much reduction in the swelling. "The physical therapist wasn't very encouraged because of the amount of radiation I'd had," she said. "My goal was to maintain the level of swelling I had and not let it get any worse"—though she thought there'd been a slight increase in swelling over the preceding year. She said, "If I dedicated an hour and a half to two hours a day to work with it, maybe it wouldn't be getting worse, I don't know. Anyway, the lymphatic massage treatment was one of the most pleasant, gentle, and relaxing things I have ever experienced."

After the regimen of lymphatic massage was completed she continued to bandage at night and to do self-massage, particularly when she noticed an episode of swelling. "At first, my husband helped with my back. We worked steadily on it for quite a while, though I still have a pocket of lymphedema there. When I didn't see improvement in my arm, I requested the pump. But the pump was not for me. It hurt and I had to dedicate so much time to it. I tried it for about a month, setting aside time every day for it. It was beginning to seem like it was ruling my life. Everything else I wanted to do—all the activities of life like school committees, programs for my children, gardening—didn't allow me time to sit and be on the pump. I decided I was not going to let it rule my life, so I gave up on it." She said she did have one patient who had used the pump with good results.

Nancy continued with self-massage and intermittently bandaged, but she didn't see any change. "It was hard," she said. "Some nights I just wanted to go to sleep with nothing on my arm." She also tried using the Reid sleeve, a type of wrap that is similar to bandages but straps onto the arm (or the leg in the case of lower-extremity lymphedema). She said, "Because I see a lot of information coming across my desk, I found out about the Reid sleeve, and the pictures made it look tolerable. I wanted to just be able to slip my arm in the sleeve and go to bed at night. It took more than six months for my insurance company to agree to pay for it. When I got the sleeve, it was enormous and not at all what I'd imagined. But, as cumbersome as it is, I do still use it at times."

She held out her arm again and fingered a silver-chain bracelet on her wrist. "I use this as a sort of gauge," she said. "There are times when the bracelet's so tight around my wrist that it leaves big dents." That day, the bracelet swung loosely. "When my arm is actively swelling I'll bandage at night and wear a Juzo sleeve during the day. When it's not a problem I use the Reid sleeve alone, though I've found that bandaging is most effective. I have discovered a new Juzo sleeve that has silicone grippers at the top. It's a lot better than the old sleeves, because it stays up. I couldn't work with the older models, but I have no trouble at all with the new one."

In her field, she encounters patients with lymphedema and refers them to physical therapy for lymphatic massage. And to those who don't have lymphedema, she talks about general precautions. She said, "It's another thing that makes me glad I know how to be of help."

At one point during our conversation she fell silent for a moment. Finally she said, "Do you know what really sort of bothers me? When I show someone my arm and they say, 'That's not so bad.' I guess it isn't that bad from the perspective of somebody else, but to me it seems so big and obvious." She lightly rubbed the edema around her elbow, then slipped back into her sweater. "I have to shop differently now. I find myself wearing sweaters to cover my arm even in the summer. I dread summer because of the heat." She sighed and continued, "I see women taking all kinds of measures to deal with their swelling, wearing gloves and sleeves and going regularly for treatments, and they don't experience as much lymphedema as I have. Maybe if I had that kind of attitude, my arm wouldn't be as swollen—I don't know."

"I do take care, however," she said. "I don't ignore my arm and I don't jeopardize its condition, but I don't let it run my life, either." When we spoke five years ago, her son was fifteen and her daughter thirteen. She continued, "Our family is just like everyone else's, I guess—we're so busy. My son has tennis at seven o'clock, my daughter has to be at school at seven forty-five. I have to be at work by eight." She laughed; it was obvious she loved doing all she did. "Now, how am I going to be able to put more time into lymphedema?"

She went on, "I guess the best thing that has come out of this last few years is my sense of living better each day. You know, in a way, that year of dealing with cancer turned out to be one of the best years of my life. I spent time with myself, and with my family, and with friends I normally never have time with. Even if I'd known ahead of time that I'd get lymphedema, I would have chosen to go through everything I did for the cancer. I've had four years of health, and four good years with my family. That's not so bad after all."

Five years after our first visit I called Nancy to see how she was doing. Over ten years had passed since she'd been treated for breast cancer. She told me, "I feel good again, though I really can't say I'll ever feel cured of it." As for her lymphedema, she said, "It's stable now and under control. It doesn't bother me much any more." She has kept active. "I work out at the gym three times a week—on the Stairmaster, on the treadmill, and with light weights." She doesn't bandage, though she wears a sleeve when she flies and wears gloves when she gardens. She said she is careful in many of the choices she makes; for instance, she doesn't get fake nails or manicures, as a precaution.

She concluded, "My arm with lymphededma is slightly larger than the other, and that means now and then I'll find a blazer or blouse that may not fit right, so I don't buy it." Her tone affirmed that she'd pretty much put cancer and lymphedema behind her.

15

CAROLYN'S STORY
USING *a* VASOPNEUMATIC PUMP

Carolyn is in her early forties. She is short, not much over five feet tall, and has curly black hair. She is a teacher's aide at a grade school, where she works with children who have learning disorders. She also tutors foreign students in English. She has an eager, alert expression, and it is hard to imagine kids being able to put much over on her.

When we met she wore a short-sleeved T-shirt. One arm was noticeably larger than the other. She wore no jewelry on that arm. A couple of years earlier, within a week of starting a new job at the school, she learned she had a recurrence of cancer. Earlier she'd gone through treatment for breast cancer. This time it had metastasized to her bones—mostly to her pelvis, but also to a spot on the top of her head and several other places. She had quit the tamoxifen the doctors had prescribed after her breast cancer because the medication, which blocks the effects of estrogen in the body, had caused her terrible hot flashes. She said, "When the cancer came back I felt real bad, as if that's what had caused it. But the doctor said the cancer would have come back anyway sometime."

She underwent chemo and radiation again, and took Taxol, which she had to discontinue because it gave her severe pain. When we visited she was on high-dose Megace. She reported that the hot flashes weren't as bad as they had been, but she still experienced water retention and weight gain. The drugs had increased her appetite.

The cancer had disappeared from everywhere except one last spot in her pelvis.

Carolyn spoke as directly about her lymphedema—which developed right after her mastectomy—as she'd spoken about her cancer. It affected her lower arm mostly but also her upper arm to a lesser degree. She asked her doctor about the swelling, but he did not seem to have any idea about what could be done. She told me, "It was the clerk at the place where I bought my breast prosthesis who told me about lymphedema. The store had pictures on the walls of people who had it really bad. Until then, I still didn't know where to get help."

Carolyn's mother bought her a Lymphapress pump. It cost three thousand dollars. Carolyn used it for four years. She said, "Every night I would sit for two hours with my arm in the pump and it would take the swelling down. But a couple of hours later my arm would swell up again." Finally, three months before our interview, she'd been referred to a lymphedema therapist who taught her drainage massage and exercises and showed her how to bandage. Carolyn continued, "She was surprised when I told her I had a pump. She asked what pressure I had it at and I told her it was at eighty millimeters. She quickly advised me, 'Set it lower. It shouldn't be any higher than thirty-five millimeters.' She was so emphatic that I set it lower even before I turned it on again." Carolyn inspected her arm and said, "It's going down now. But the therapist said it might have weighed fifteen pounds more than the other before I started treatment."

She wrapped the fingers of her unaffected arm around the wrist of the arm with lymphedema; they came within half an inch of meeting. She said, "Before, I couldn't get my fingers within an inch and a half of coming together." She also had lymphedema in her trunk and chest, and in front of her armpit. She indicated where in the armpit the swelling had occurred and said that it had gone away since she'd begun treatment.

She said, "After all the trouble I've had in the last four years, I'm real good about massaging and bandaging every night. And I do the exercises and then rewrap before I go to bed. I love this regimen, because I don't have to spend hours on the machine anymore. But a couple of times I've used the machine when it was hot and my arm was really swollen." She rarely eats anything with salt in it anymore. "And I really am careful to drink lots of water," she said. "Water really helps keep down the swelling in my arm. I notice the difference when I don't drink enough. In fact, last weekend I got some sort of bug and I had diarrhea. I got dehydrated and my arms really swelled up. So I'm convinced drinking water is real important for me."

Carolyn also started going to an herbalist. She said, "She's teaching me that my body is a healing machine. She's teaching me to think positively and not to associate every little ache and pain with cancer. And I'm learning to tell the cancer to go away." She laughs. "I say, 'Cancer, you're not welcome here. You've got to go.' "

She continued, "The herbalist has taught me to pretend I am on a cliff and if I make one misstep I'll fall down a thousand-foot drop. And I picture grabbing every crack, every hold I can, to keep going, just like I do to keep away the cancer."

16

EXERCISING *with* LYMPHEDEMA

We take it for granted that exercise is good for us. But do we do it? Many of us probably don't exercise as much or as regularly as we should. We may take a stab at it now and then, perhaps joining a health club or making a pact with our best friend, but, honestly, how many of us follow through?

If ever there was a time to find an exercise program and stick with it, that time is now, when you're recovering from breast cancer and its treatment and starting treatment for lymphedema. Former patients of Gwen's often stop by her clinic for a visit, sometimes years after treatment, and they tell her that the single most important factor in successfully keeping their lymphedema under control has been following a regular exercise program.

Overall Benefits of Exercise

We all know that exercise offers many important health benefits, including cancer prevention, decreased risk of heart disease and type-2 diabetes, and weight management. Exercise can also help in the recovery from cancer. Research shows it can improve outcomes after surgery and chemotherapy, promote a high level of independence, make patients less fatigued and nauseated, and decrease depression.[1] The American Institute for Cancer Research reports, "Dietary choices, together with exercise and a healthy weight, could prevent three to four million cancer cases worldwide each year."[2] One study showed that women who exercise for four hours a week have a 37 percent lower incidence of breast cancer than sedentary women.[3] Women who exercise regularly generally have a lower percentage of body fat. Body fat generates more estrogen in the system, which may put some women at higher risk for breast cancer. Studies also suggest that exercise can be helpful in decreasing the risk of breast cancer recurrence. Finally, obesity, as discussed earlier in the book, puts a woman at higher risk for developing lymphedema.[4,5,6]

If all these reasons aren't enough to motivate us to start exercising and keep at it, Gwen reports that in her experience the people who best manage their lymphedema have established and stuck with a regular exercise program. Before you begin, though, a word of caution: Some exercises, particularly if they are not carried out in moderation, can actually worsen lymphedema. Gwen remembers a patient who had been protecting her arm for two years after breast cancer in fear of developing lymphedema. She was advised by her surgeon to exercise it actively. She followed her doctor's orders and developed lymphedema, which has never completely resolved.

A comprehensive lymphedema treatment program includes several types of specialized exercises, which are described later in the chapter. First, though, let's talk about how to get more exercise in general. One way is to incorporate physical activity into your daily habits. Here are some quick suggestions for doing that:

* Park at the far end of the parking lot, or park several blocks away from your destination.

* Take the stairs instead of the elevator.

* At work, take short, frequent breaks throughout the day to move around. Walk to a rest room at the other end of the building rather than one right next to your office. Walk to a coworker's office rather than e-mailing or phoning her or him.

* During sports events such as soccer or football games, get up and walk around.

✳ Fill your grocery bags only halfway (it is better anyway to decrease the amount of weight you carry) and then make more trips into your house to carry them in. Also, walk that empty grocery cart back to the store.

✳ Instead of driving, walk or bike to do some of your errands.

✳ Drink eight to ten glasses of water every day. Besides keeping you well hydrated, doing so will keep you moving as you frequently visit the bathroom.

✳ Plan family outings that involve physical activities like hiking, tennis, or cycling.

✳ Have fun! Dance around as you listen to your favorite music. Engage your children or grandchildren in playful activities.

Special Exercises for Lymphedema Treatment

As we've mentioned, all comprehensive therapy and rehabilitation programs for lymphedema incorporate special exercises.[7] The exercises fall into several different categories, four of which we'll cover in this chapter. Each category has a different treatment goal.

1. *Lymph-drainage exercises.* These are simple mobility exercises performed in a specific sequence to pump the fluid through the lymphatic pathways, away from congested areas and into areas of improved drainage.

2. *Stretching and flexibility exercises.* These exercises help achieve mobility, which is the ability to move muscles and joints through their full range of motion. *Flexibility* refers to the degree of normal motion, and *stretching* refers to the process of elongating muscles and other soft tissues.[8] After breast cancer surgery, women may experience tightness in the pectoral area (chest) and armpit and decreased range of motion in the shoulder. This loss of mobility may interfere with normal lymph or venous drainage from the arm.[9]

3. *Strengthening and toning exercises.* These exercises build the muscles' power for the purpose of improving endurance and capability of performance. The stronger the muscle, the better able it is to perform without overexertion or fatigue. It has been reported that progressive resistance training (pushing and pulling with a light weight or stretchy band) can increase lymphatic flow.[8] Resistance exercise has also proven beneficial in the prevention of osteoporosis.

4. *Aerobic exercises.* Dr. Kenneth Cooper defines this as "exercise which demands large quantities of oxygen for prolonged periods to force the body to improve those systems responsible for transportation of oxygen."[10] More simply, this means exercising at a pace that increases your heart and breathing rates, which is usually accomplished by using the large muscles.

Examples of each of these types of exercise and instructions for how to do them are provided later in the chapter.

Goals of Exercise as a Part of Lymphedema Treatment

The reasons for exercising are varied. The primary goals of exercising to help treat lymphedema are to move lymph fluid and to reduce swelling. More specifically, exercise should [11]

* *pump the muscles to move lymph from the congested area into an area where it can more easily drain.* As with lymphatic massage, the first emphasis is to clear the trunk. Only after the trunk is cleared do you exercise to drain your arm.

* *increase mobility of the shoulder girdle and spine.* The book *Physical Therapy for the Cancer Patient* reports that a common problem after breast cancer is decreased mobility and strength in the involved arm, particularly the shoulder girdle (which encompasses the shoulder blade, collarbone, shoulder, and upper arm).[12]

✳ *increase muscle strength and tone.* Decreased strength can occur in the arm after breast cancer. Most often, diminution in strength is caused by disuse, pain, imbalances in posture, or fear of using the arm. Loss of strength can happen rapidly. If you have had a mastectomy, the muscles of the shoulder girdle and shoulder blade may weaken if you unconsciously guard the area and do not move your muscles naturally. Or the development of scar tissue can make your shoulder pull forward, which can result in improper posture. The potential for scarring increases if you've had reconstruction using your own tissue. In this procedure, the muscles are rearranged, leading to the potential for even more scar tissue and greater muscle imbalance, which eventually can lead to pain in the trunk. It is important to overcome these tendencies and to restore muscle balance in the upper trunk. Strengthening the area may allow you to do more activity without triggering the lymphatic response.

✳ *improve circulation.* One method of improving lymph flow is to pump the blood vessels, an action that can stimulate a stretch reflex in the lymph vessels, causing them to contract and move lymph fluid.

✳ *improve body awareness and promote a sense of general well-being.* Regular aerobic exercise can cause the body to secrete hormones called *endorphins* that have been shown to be associated with feelings of euphoria and well-being. Endorphins are also powerful analgesics. It is believed that endorphins can be released even with exercise of relatively mild intensity.[10]

Guidelines for Exercising with Lymphedema

If you have a set of bandages or a compression garment, wear either of them during exercise. Bandages in particular increase pressure against the skin during the workout. The higher pressure, coupled with the contraction of the muscles, encourages the lymph to move.

If you want to wear a compression garment during exercise, remember that its specific purpose is to *maintain* a reduction in swelling, not necessarily to reduce it.

Some of you may lack access to complete decongestive therapy and/or bandaging treatment. If so, the exercises outlined below can still be carried out with some benefit to lymph flow.[13] Learning to breathe using your diaphragm and belly will stimulate lymph circulation in your trunk (see Chapter 7). Your muscles can act as a pump against the lymph vessels, and your circulatory system will be pumping as well. Exercising without bandages or garments is better than not exercising at all. A note of caution: Do not substitute Ace wraps for short-stretch lymphedema bandages. Ace bandages are not intended for use in lymphedema as they do not provide enough pressure to move lymph. They may even cause an interruption in lymph flow. (See Chapter 12.)

As for how much exercise to do and how fast to do it, use your arm as a monitor. If it swells, cut back some on your level of activity, and build up more slowly. The program we suggest is not a recipe that fits everyone. No program does. In order to gain the most benefit you'll need to modify it to meet your individual needs. For example, if you have a back problem or shoulder problem for which you are already doing exercises, you'll need to consider that in your regimen. There may be any number of factors that do not allow you to carry out all the exercises suggested in this chapter. Please get the input or advice of a trained therapist before you begin. The program we provide should be taken as an example of one you may want to consider. It is not all-inclusive, nor are the exercises the only effective ones. Many routines can prove successful.

As always, use common sense. If you overdo it, your arm may swell a bit more, but don't worry—you will probably be able to quickly reduce the swelling by following the easy steps we outlined earlier: First, drink a large glass of water, then elevate your arm in a passive position (prop it up while fully relaxing the muscles of the arm), do some diaphragmatic breathing, and back off from using the arm for a day. If you have had an eventful day with lots of physical activity, let up on your exercises a bit. If you are feeling fatigued or tired, don't push yourself; take that into account and adjust your routine. Your program should not be rigid, but flexible and persistent. If you notice swelling that does not resolve with conservative measures within a few days, you might want to consider seeing a lymphedema therapist.

Here are a few more guiding principles to keep in mind as you design your exercise program:

* Be sure to consult with your doctor before starting any regular exercise. If you experience any problems once you've begun exercising, stop your routine and talk to your doctor.

* During exercise use some form of compression on your arm if it's available, especially as you're beginning a new exercise program.

* Start very slowly. Perform few repetitions and wait until the next day to see how your arm has responded.

* Gradually increase the repetitions, always using your arm as a guide to how much you can do. Always use low resistance.

* Make sure to continue a smooth breathing pattern throughout the exercise routine. Overcome the tendency to hold your breath. Relax your abdominal muscles and practice breathing into your belly.

* Use proper posture to open up all channels of possible fluid movement and to facilitate a good breathing pattern. Here's what we mean by proper posture: The feet should be well planted to create a stable base, and the knees unlocked. The buttocks should be lightly tucked but not clenched. Pull the belly button in toward the spine. Keep your chest up, shoulders relaxed and dropped down, head back and squarely over the shoulders. The trick of imagining a string pulling upward from the crown of the head really works.

* Always move slowly and deliberately, being aware of which muscles you are using. Concentrate on the movement. Pause between repetitions.

❋ *Never* cause pain. The old adage "No pain, no gain" is not accurate. You should never experience any significant discomfort while you exercise (other than the discomfort and bulk of all those bandages).

❋ Keep yourself well hydrated during exercise by drinking several glasses of water.

When You Should *Not* Exercise

Avoid exercise or stop exercising under the following circumstances:

❋ When you are ill with a fever

❋ If you experience chest pain

❋ If you experience sudden shortness of breath or unusual fatigue

❋ If you have recurring leg pain or cramps

❋ If you experience an acute onset of nausea during exercise

❋ If you feel disoriented or confused

❋ If you have suffered recent bone, back, or neck pain that is not relieved with rest

❋ If you have an irregular heartbeat[14]

The rest of the chapter outlines a regimen of special exercises that will aid in the treatment of lymphedema.

Lymph-Drainage Exercises

While it is best for people with lymphedema to follow a comprehensive exercise program, the first and most important exercises for them are the lymph-drainage exercises. The ones outlined here are the ones Gwen uses at her clinic; many other good exercise programs follow the same general principles but may be slightly different. If you have any trouble doing any of the exercises exactly as they are described, just modify them so you can do them. For example, it's not necessary to acheive the strongest possible muscle contraction; just make it strong enough so you can feel it. The idea is to simply contract the muscles in the sequence presented here: Start with the trunk, then move to the neck, then the shoulder, and finally end at the hand.

We recommend repeating each exercise two or three times. If you feel like you want to do more, repeat the sequence of exercises again; do not just do more repetitions of each one. Before each exercise, start with four or five slow abdominal breaths.

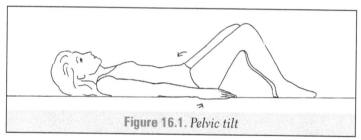

Figure 16.1. *Pelvic tilt*

1. *Pelvic tilt.* Lie on your back with your knees bent and feet flat on the bed or floor. Pull up and in with the abdominal muscles, tilting the pelvis and flattening the lower back into the bed or floor.

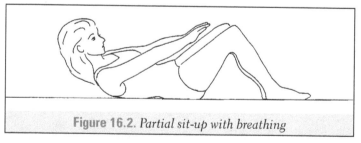

Figure 16.2. *Partial sit-up with breathing*

2. *Partial sit-up with breathing.* Again, lie on your back with your knees bent and feet flat on the bed or floor. Breathe into your belly. As you exhale, lift your head and shoulders, just barely clearing the floor, and reach forward with your hands. Be careful not to cause pain or strain in your neck.

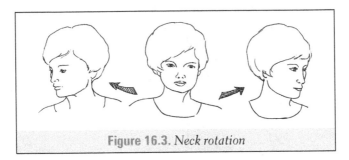

Figure 16.3. *Neck rotation*

3. *Neck rotation.* Turn your head slowly to the right as you inhale and count to five. Return to the center as you exhale. Repeat to the left.

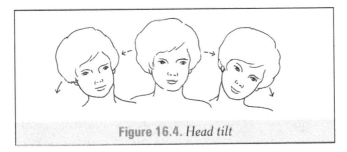

Figure 16.4. *Head tilt*

4. *Head tilt.* Tilt your head to the right, allowing your ear to drop toward your shoulder. Maintain this position for a count of five, then slowly bring your head back to the center. Repeat to the other side.

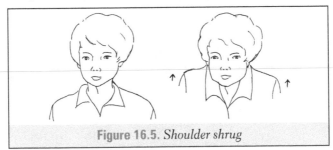

Figure 16.5. *Shoulder shrug*

5. *Shoulder shrug.* Lift both shoulders toward your ears as you breathe in. Then return to a relaxed position. Next, pull your shoulders down as far as possible; then return to a relaxed position.

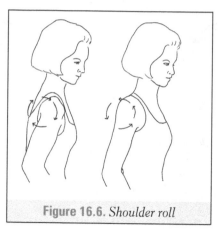

Figure 16.6. *Shoulder roll*

6. *Shoulder roll.* Lift the shoulders up toward the ears, then rotate them back and drop them down, making a smooth, continuous, circular motion.

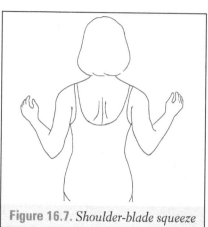

Figure 16.7. *Shoulder-blade squeeze*

7. *Shoulder-blade squeeze.* Bend your elbows to about ninety degrees. Keeping your elbows close to your body, pull them toward the center of your back, squeezing the shoulder blades together.

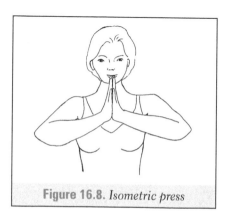

Figure 16.8. *Isometric press*

8. *Isometric hand press.* Place the palms of your hands together, with your elbows bent and arms at shoulder or chest level. Push your palms together firmly while breathing in to a count of four; then relax and breathe out to a count of four.

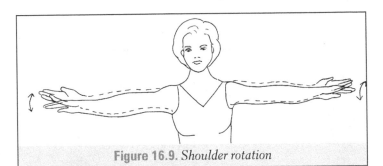

Figure 16.9. *Shoulder rotation*

9. *Shoulder rotation.* With the arms extended at shoulder height, rotate the palms outward slowly, so they are facing upward. Then rotate the arms inward so the palms are facing back. If you have shoulder problems and it is difficult for you to do the motion at shoulder height, just raise your arms as far as is comfortable.

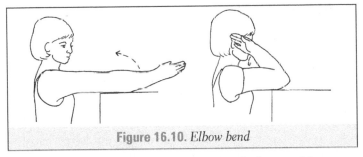

Figure 16.10. *Elbow bend*

10. *Elbow bend.* Sit with your arm extended on a table or counter at shoulder height. Again, if this is a problem for your shoulder, just do the exercise with your arm at your side. Bend your elbow, bringing your hand toward your shoulder. Return to the start position.

11. *Wrist circle.* Make a fist and rotate it in small circles, keeping the movement isolated to the wrist only. Rotate first in one direction, then in the other.

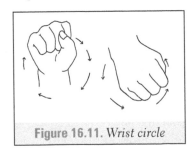

Figure 16.11. *Wrist circle*

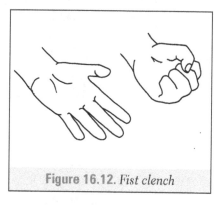

Figure 16.12. *Fist clench*

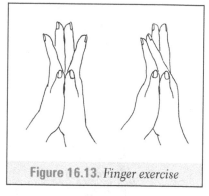

Figure 16.13. *Finger exercise*

12. *Fist clench.* Open your hands and spread your fingers apart. Then slowly clench each hand to make a fist. Hold for three seconds, then relax.

13. *Finger exercise.* Hold your hands in front of you, palms together. Separate matching pairs of fingers by opening them away from each other, one pair at a time; then reverse the sequence. As an additional exercise, hold the fingers together as you move each pair from side to side.

14. *Breathing.* Practice belly breathing (see Chapter 7).

After you complete the lymph-drainage exercises, it is a good idea to lie down and relax for a few minutes (or longer) with your arm supported and elevated on a pillow.

Stretching and Flexibility Exercises

As mentioned earlier, lack of flexibility in the shoulder girdle and trunk after breast cancer can be caused by scar tissue or tightness in the connective tissue. This tissue responds best to low-force, long-duration stretching.[15] Tightness can also be caused by holding the arm in a protected position and not moving it freely. If your arm is immobilized, it can quickly stiffen up, which can contribute to additional problems. Stretching exercises can restore flexibility to the areas affected by breast cancer and its treatment. (See also the discussion in Chapter 10 on massage and stretching techniques for scar tissue, cording, and myofascial release.)

As you do the exercises outlined in this section, try stretching just short of the point at which your muscle, scar tissue, or joint feels pain, then holding that position for several seconds. Stretching should be done slowly and with deliberation, from a well-aligned position, taking care to maintain a smooth, even breathing pattern throughout. One trick is to hold a stretch position for three or four slow breaths while imagining that you are breathing oxygen into the area and releasing tension as you exhale.

Hundreds of stretching and flexibility routines exist besides those presented here. Many excellent books give good information on stretching. Two that seem very user-friendly are *Stretching* (20th anniversary edition), by Bob and Jean Anderson, and *Essential Guide to Stretching*, by Chrissie Gallagher-Mundy (see Recommended Reading). Though the emphasis in the exercises we've included here is mostly on the health of the shoulder and shoulder girdle, you will nonetheless reap other benefits by incorporating a stretching program for your entire body, such as these books recommend, into your exercise regimen.

Modify the program as you need to, and remember, never force your body or cause unnecessary pain.

Stretches for the Shoulder

1. *Cane exercise.* Use a broomstick or cane. Hold it in front of your chest with your palms facing away from the body. Lift the stick up over your head, and then lower it so that it is behind your head. (If you can't bring the stick fully over your head, just lift it up as far as you can.) Hold this position for three slow breaths, then return to the start position.

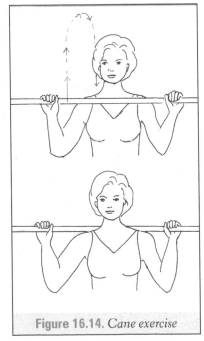

Figure 16.14. *Cane exercise*

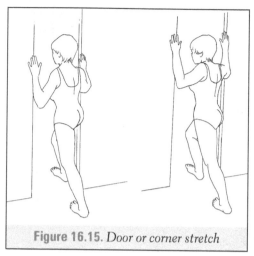
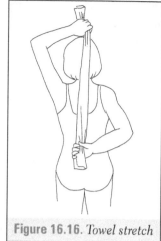

Figure 16.15. *Door or corner stretch*

Figure 16.16. *Towel stretch*

2. *Door or corner stretch.* Stand facing a corner or open doorway. Raise your elbows, keeping them below your shoulders, and rest your forearms against the two walls or against the sides of the doorframe. Lean your entire body forward, so that your upper torso is in front of your arms and you feel the stretch in your chest. Maintain the stretch for fifteen to twenty seconds. You can vary this exercise and stretch different parts of the chest by gradually raising your arms higher.

3. *Towel stretch.* Hold each end of a towel behind your back, with one arm behind your lower back and the other arm overhead. Pull the towel up and down as if you were drying your back.

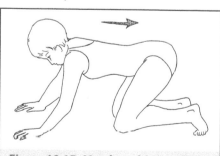

Figure 16.17. *Hands-and-knees stretch*

4. *Hands-and-knees stretch.* Rest on your hands and knees with your hands slightly in front of your shoulders. Rock back toward your heels, stretching your shoulders.

Strengthening and Toning Exercises

Gradually you can add exercises to your program that include some resistance, in the form of either a Theraband (see below) or light hand weights. Studies have demonstrated that strengthening exercises do not seem to increase lymphedema in women after breast cancer if the patient uses low resistance in the beginning and progresses gradually and slowly to higher resistance.[16] As with all exercise, it is important to monitor your body's response to the activity and modify it accordingly the next time you do it.

If you do add some form of resistance to your workout, start slowly. Begin with a low resistance and a few repetitions, and gradually increase over several months, especially if you have not previously exercised regularly.

The Theraband is a stretchy elastic band color-coded for different levels of resistance. Using it increases the workload, helping to build muscle tone and strength. If you want to use weights, start with one or two pounds, and, again, gradually increase the number of repetitions and the amount of weight over several months. Always monitor your arm for increased swelling. If swelling persists for more than twenty-four hours after a workout, you need to decrease the number of repetitions or the amount of weight you're using.[17] Bonnie Lasinski, a lymphedema therapist, writes, "The important thing to consider is whether you feel good after the exercise and how your affected limb reacts.... You must also consider your level of daily activity and modify accordingly."[18]

There are several areas to focus on when doing strengthening exercises after breast cancer. The first is the shoulder area. Gwen finds that many women have lost strength in their upper back and around their shoulder blades. Second, all the muscle groups of the arm can benefit from strengthening so the arm will not be overloaded or fatigued by the activities of daily living. Another benefit of working the arm muscles with light resistance is that doing so pumps the muscles, which assists with lymph drainage. Especially important are the muscles that lie along the path of alternative lymphatic drainage, such as the deltoid, which lies over the top of the shoulder, and the triceps, which is in the back of the upper arm. The third area that *all* people can benefit from strengthening is the abdominal muscles. Remember to avoid contracting the abdominal muscles continually for long periods of time, as doing so prevents you from belly breathing.

It would be overwhelming to cover all the strenghtening exercises you could incorporate into your routine. Instead, we have included a few examples of the types of exercises that Gwen has used with her patients. Since each exercise program for lymphedema needs to be individualized, consider seeking the advice of a trained therapist to evaluate your specific needs and to establish a program designed to meet them.

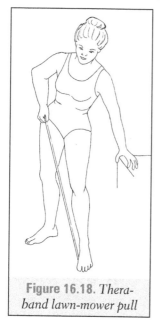

Figure 16.18. *Theraband lawn-mower pull*

Using a Theraband or Rubber Tubing

1. *Lawn-mower pull.* Stand on one end of the Theraband and wrap the other end around your hand on the involved side. Bend over slightly, perhaps holding on to a counter or table. Pull your arm back as if you were starting a lawn mower. Move deliberately rather than jerking. Repeat five to seven times.

2. *Chest pull.* Hold each end of the band at chest height and with your hands about shoulder width apart. Pull out to the side, extending your arms outward while squeezing your

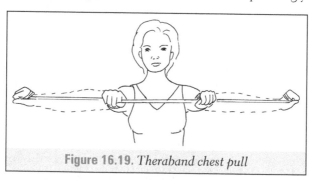

Figure 16.19. *Theraband chest pull*

shoulder blades together. Make sure your wrists don't bend; the hands should follow the movement of the arms. Repeat five to seven times.

Using Light Weights

Start these exercises with one-pound weights and build up to a maximum of three pounds.

1. *Arms out to side.* Start by standing with a small weight in each hand and your arms hanging at your sides; then raise your arms out and up to shoulder height. Keep your palms

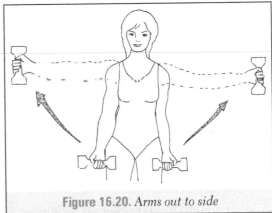

Figure 16.20. *Arms out to side*

facing forward the whole time and keep your shoulders down. Hold this position for five seconds, then slowly lower your arms. Repeat five to seven times.

2. *Reaching to the ceiling.* Lie on your back with knees bent and feet flat on the floor. Holding a weight in the hand of your involved arm, extend the arm toward the ceiling, directly above your shoulder. Bend your elbow so that the weight is lowered toward the shoulder of

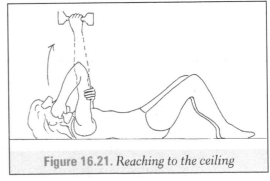

Figure 16.21. *Reaching to the ceiling*

the same arm, and then raise the weight toward the ceiling again. Make sure your upper arm stays more or less vertical rather than moving with the forearm; the goal here is to work mostly the triceps, which requires moving only the forearm in this exercise. If you want, you can support your upper arm with the other hand, as illustrated. Repeat five to seven times.

Aerobic Exercises

Aerobic exercise can serve you in many ways. The movement of the exercise coupled with the deep breathing it requires can cause a reduction in swelling by increasing lymph flow and improving the fluid balance in your body.[16] In addition, as your cardiovascular system works harder to pump blood during aerobic exercise, it stimulates the lymph vessels that run alongside the blood vessels. This action enhances lymph flow. The lymphatic system is stimulated by both the pumping action of the blood vessels and the pumping action of the muscles, so anything you do to improve your circulatory system will be helpful for the lymphatic system.

Before you launch into an aerobic exercise program, here's a short list of things to consider:

1. Be careful not to exercise in the heat of the day. Exercise when it's cool, in the morning or in the evening.

2. If you are using a machine indoors, exercise in a cool, air-conditioned place.

3. Don't choose an activity that strains or jars your body, or one that could lead to injury.

4. If you have a support garment or bandages, wear them while exercising.

5. As with all activities, monitor yourself closely for twenty-four hours after exercising, watching for any of the warning signs that fluid may be building up.

6. If you notice any symptoms of swelling, elevate your arm, drink some water, and modify the exercise for the next time.

Consult your therapist about which specific sports and exercises may be best for you. However, you're more likely to have greater—and continued—success if you choose activities that you enjoy. If you dislike organized exercise classes or getting into water, try walking or biking. Not everyone is up for the elliptical trainer or stair stepper. The activity just needs to mildly increase your heart rate. With any type of aerobic exercise, remember to do some simple warm-up exercises before beginning and some cool-down exercises afterward.

A good goal to work toward is exercising thirty to forty minutes per day, six to seven days a week. The time can be divided into separate increments if that works better for you; the cumulative minutes are what is most important. You could take a ten-minute walk during lunch, another ten-minute walk after work, and add a ten- to fifteen-minute bike ride.

As you exercise, take your pulse at your wrist or neck while at rest and again at different times during the workout. General guidelines are to stay within 60 and 80 percent of your maximum heart rate. To calculate, subtract your age from 220 (the resulting number is your maximum heart rate); then multiply that number by 60 percent and 80 percent. Your target range is between those two numbers. If your arm tends to swell when you exercise, Gwen strongly suggests staying at the 60 percent level or below.

Water aerobics, water walking, and swimming are especially good activities as they take pressure off the weight-bearing joints. The rippling of water over the skin can cause some stimulation of the superficial lymphatics. The hydrostatic pressure provided by the water helps to minimize swelling by supplying compression to the affected body part. For this reason, Dr. Judith Casley-Smith recommends scuba diving for lymphedema patients.[19] For even better results some people find it helpful to wear an old support garment during swimming or pool exercises. Finally, moving in water helps to loosen up the shoulder. Check with the recreation centers or pools in your community to see what types of water-exercise programs are available.

Walking is another great activity. All you need is a good pair of shoes and a safe place to walk. The American Heart Association recommends walking at least ten thousand steps each day.[20] That's approximately four to five miles, depending on your stride length. Again, as with any exercise program, it is important to start at a lower level and gradually work up to your goals. Pedometers, small devices that are worn at the waistband and that measure how far you walk, have become very popular. They typically cost less than thirty dollars. The nice thing about a pedometer is that you can put it on in the morning so that it tracks *all* your activities—walking at the grocery store, around the house, from the car, etc. Some people are surprised by how much they actually walk in a day over and above a thirty- or forty-minute structured walk.

Besides being an important part of a lymphedema treatment plan, aerobic exercise is also a realistic way to help lose weight and keep it off. As we have discussed throughout this book, obesity is a contributing factor to an increased risk for both breast cancer and lymphedema. Regular exercise is a critical part of an effective weight-loss and weight-maintenance program.

Though a lot of aerobic exercises require no more equipment than a good pair of sports shoes, there is one apparatus that promotes both aerobic fitness and upper-body movement. It is called a UBE, or upper-body exerciser, and it is like a stationary bike for the arms. Gwen's physical therapy facility has a UBE arm, as do some health clubs and gyms. With bandages on the arm, Gwen starts the patient with one to two minutes on the machine, set to zero resistance. If your gym has a UBE, you can do the same thing. Warm up to it, though, and wear your bandages. Remember, it is better to err on the side of less.

Finally, be cautious of working with trainers at health clubs. They may be unfamiliar with lymphedema and may be overzealous.

Other Exercises

Besides those we've already discussed, a wide variety of exercises can help lymphedema patients. The book *Essential Exercises for Breast Cancer Survivors*, by Amy Halverstadt and Andrea Leonard, outlines

exercises that can be done right after surgery as well as guidelines for
developing a long-term exercise program. This section describes a
few more exercises that might be suitable and enjoyable for you. For
publication details about any of the books mentioned in this section, see Recommended Reading, located at the back of the book.

Ethafoam Roller

Gwen has found it useful to work with an Ethafoam roller, a firm,
Styrofoam-like cylinder four to six inches in diameter. You can lie on
your back with the roll under your spine and do some breathing, balancing, arm movements, and opposing movements with arm and leg
(Figure 16.22). You can roll from side to side. These types of exercises have proven effective in orthopedic situations. They may also

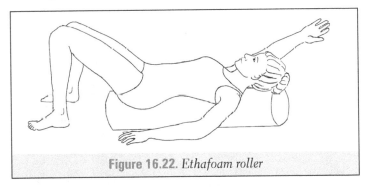

Figure 16.22. Ethafoam roller

help to mobilize the spine and the muscles alongside the spine.
Theoretically, this can influence the collateral lymph vessels, which
carry fluid across the watersheds to the healthy quadrant. They also
help to mobilize the ribs, assist with improved breathing patterns,
and promote improved posture.

Some therapists recommend using a "noodle," a six-foot-long
Styrofoam roll that is used as a swimming-pool flotation device. It is
only about three inches wide and is made of softer material, but it
can be used in place of the Ethafoam roller if you cannot find one of
those. Another alternative is to roll up a beach towel very tightly, so
it is three to four inches in diameter, and then wrap tape around it.

Gwen relates an experience with one of her first lymphedema
patients. She came in the week before Gwen was scheduled to go to

her first lymphedema training program. Gwen didn't know about lymphatic massage or any other treatment techniques for lymphedema, but she did know about neck and back dysfunctions and was familiar with muscle spasms. Gwen plunged into treatment of the woman's musculoskeletal dysfunctions and put her on an Ethafoam roller. After working with the roller for several minutes, teaching the patient some diaphragm breathing, and giving her some postural pointers, the two women looked at the patient's arm and were shocked to see that it had visibly decreased in size. What Gwen knows now is that they had cleared out her trunk to create room for the fluid to drain into. The tight muscles along the patient's spine, her stiff and rounded upper back, and her poor breathing patterns were contributing to blockage of lymph flow, and working on these issues helped her immediately. Ever since then, Gwen has been using the roller with lymphedema patients.

Therapy Ball or Gymnastic Ball

Another exercise device is the therapy ball or gymnastic ball, a large, strong ball that comes in different sizes. It is a fun and versatile tool

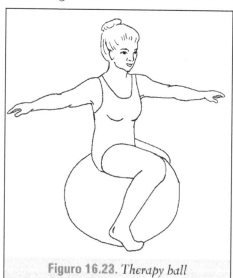

Figuro 16.23. *Therapy ball*

that can be used for a variety of exercises. You can sit on it (Figure 16.23), lie on your back and stretch over it, or lie over it on your stomach. You can use it for various stretching, strengthening, and stabilization programs. It is especially good for developing abdominal and back strength. You can use both the ball and the Ethafoam roller at home on a regular basis and they can be purchased through a medical supply company or through your health-care provider's physical therapy department. Since therapy balls are currently popular for use in Pilates-style exercise programs, many retailers that sell sports equipment also now carry them. The large balls available in toy stores are usually not strong enough for these exercises and should not be used. As always, consult with a therapist to help you find the most appropriate—and safest—exercises for your situation.

Tai Chi, Yoga, and Other Fun Activities

Many lymphedema patients have found it helpful to practice tai chi or qigong (pronounced "chee-gong"). Traditional exercises from China, both incorporate slow, deliberate movements that focus on breathing and alignment. In Chapter 22, Feather's story illustrates how qigong has helped her.

Yoga, too, can be a wonderful help, with its focus on breathing (called _pranayama_), posture, tuning in to the body, and being with the movement. There are many different types of yoga. If you are interested in pursuing yoga, experiment with different classes to find a teacher and style that "fits" for you. We suggest trying to find a teacher who is experienced in working with people who have health issues. A good yoga teacher will give you a specific program of poses and breathing individualized for your needs. As with all exercises, it is important to start slowly and progress very gradually. With yoga, it is not the end posture that is most important; rather, it is the process of paying attention to what is happening with your body and finding your own limits. The intent is never to cause pain. While it may be better to learn yoga from a teacher instead of a video or book, there are some good yoga books available, including _Yoga for Women_, by Paddy O'Brien, _The Healing Path of Yoga_, by Nischala Joy Devi, _Restorative Yoga_, by Judith Lassiter, P.T., and _The Healing Power of Movement_, by Lisa Hoffman.

Another type of yoga, Laughter Yoga, combines deep yoga breathing, gentle stretching, and staged laughter that quickly converts to the real thing when practiced in a group. A physician who believes that laughter is the best medicine, Dr. Madan Kataria, founder of Laughter Yoga, travels the globe spreading his passionate message that "one must laugh or else fall sick." There are Laughter Yoga clubs throughout the world.

NIA (neuromuscular integrative action) is another exercise program that is growing in popularity. NIA promotes itself as an "innovative, aerobic, mind-body healing modality that incorporates a diverse blend of movements, including tai chi, aikido, dance, yoga, Feldenkrais, and Alexander technique." NIA classes are available at some athletic clubs, community centers, and other healing centers. Many classes are designed specifically to accommodate women before, during, and after breast cancer.

Dance can be wonderful exercise. Belly dancing, tap dancing, ballet—anything that gets you moving and keeps you moving is an excellent choice. Saskia Thiadens, R.N., president of the National Lymphedema Network, recommends a videotape by Sherry Lebed-Davis called *Focus on Healing Through Movement and Dance for the Breast Cancer Survivor.* Lebed-Davis also has written a book on dance and movement therapy, *Thriving after Breast Cancer.* One word of caution about dancing: Gwen remembers a patient who developed a little swelling in her arm after an evening of square dancing. Swinging her partner and doing do-si-do's were a little more vigorous than her arm could handle. As always, monitor your body's reaction to an activity, and modify accordingly. Don't overdo it. Start slowly and progress gradually. Follow the general guidelines for exercise listed earlier in the chapter. We recommend that you wear bandages or a support garment during any activity. Overexercising, even if you're doing gentle activities like qigong, tai chi, or yoga, can cause an increase of fluid, which is what you want to avoid. Don't stop your qigong, don't stop square dancing, don't stop doing anything that gets you moving. Let your arm tell you what's enough. Pay attention. If you need to, slow down, wear a compression sleeve, skip a day or two—but keep trying and keep moving.

In the past several years dragon-boat racing has become popular. There are many teams made up of breast cancer survivors who compete all over the world. Dragon boats are long, narrow boats, usually decorated with the head of a dragon, that hold several passengers who paddle to move the boat. A 2000 article in the *Journal of Surgical Oncology* challenged the idea that vigorous exercise for the upper body is contraindicated for women after axillary lymph node dissection because it can contribute to lymphedema. The researchers found that while training for a world-championship dragon-boat race only two women in the study, both of whom had preexisting lymphedema, developed a small increase in swelling; none of the other women developed swelling. They concluded that strenuous upper-body exercise may not cause lymphedema or worsen preexisting lymphedema.[21] (It is important to note that these women had a very structured training program that included stretching, strengthening, and aerobic exercises.) The study both validates how valuable a progressive exercise program can be in avoiding swelling and reinforces the recommendation that everyone should prepare themselves with stretching and strengthening for whatever activity they choose. Gwen has worked with many women who participate in dragon-boat racing to help them design an exercise program specific to their individual needs. She has found that these women get great personal pride and satisfaction from participating in this activity, as well as achieving higher levels of physical fitness than they had even before cancer.

You now have some idea of what you can do to take care of your lymphedema. No more procrastinating. No more unfulfilled promises. Start today. Find a friend to exercise with, pick an activity that you'd both enjoy, begin slowly, and gradually increase your activity level. Set yourself up to be successful. After six months you will see real benefits.

In the next chapter Anita highlights the results of her treatment program. She follows a common-sense regimen that incorporates some ideas of her own. You may want to consider it when designing yours.

17

ANITA'S STORY
a COMMITTED FOCUS YIELDS RESULTS

Anita was diagnosed with breast cancer about seven years ago. She had been an oncology nurse for many years before that. Her demeanor was warm; one would feel she'd be comforting to have as a nurse. In our first meeting she told me, "I learned that the view of cancer from a patient's perspective is a lot different from that of a nurse's. For sixteen years I had administered the same drugs I knew I'd be taking for my own cancer. It was amazing to be on the other side. It's so predictable when you're on the medical end of it. You do surgery, then chemotherapy, and, if the cancer comes back, maybe more treatment, then hospice, and...." Her voice trailed off. "I soon realized that wasn't the progression I intended for myself. I'll admit it was a very difficult time for me."

She continued, "As a nurse, I knew what worked and what didn't work. I knew the risks, including the risk of lymphedema. But, in a way, knowing is not really much help. Until you go through it, you don't know how it will feel to *you*."

Her arm and hand were covered with a compression sleeve. The arm with lymphedema was slim, appearing no different in size and shape from her other one. After her cancer diagnosis she underwent a mastectomy and four sessions of chemotherapy, but she did not receive radiation treatments. "During treatment," she said, "I had two goals: to get rid of the cancer, and to guard against lymphedema."

Though doctors at the time were beginning to be more informed about lymphedema, when Anita spoke with her surgeon about the condition he told her that if swelling didn't develop right after surgery, "it wasn't really considered lymphedema." She had swelling in her chest after surgery due to bleeding, but as she healed it went away.

"I went to work on a plan to restore my health," she said. "I wanted to get my arm mobility back and I wanted to expedite healing, so I started a program of gentle exercise." She had always been pretty active, but she enrolled in a beginners' aerobics class while she was still in chemotherapy. She said she could manage the class about half the time, when she wasn't too sick or fatigued from the chemo. All through chemo she had no changes in her involved arm, but she knew enough not to allow any IV needles to be inserted there. It was while Anita was on vacation, nine months after treatment, that she experienced a sudden swelling in her arm. She and her husband had made a four-hour flight to Chicago to visit relatives, and she didn't know any precautions to take while flying. The day after they arrived, her lower arm and her hand swelled.

She said, "I really got worried, wondering if I should call my doctor, if I should go home, stay, or what. I thought if I could get home and get back to exercising and swimming, I might be able to help it. It was really frightening. Anyway, I decided to ride out the week of vacation and try a couple things I thought might help. The muscle in my lower arm was sore, so I tried putting heat on it. I know now that wasn't the thing to do. And I tried raising my arm on a pillow. The swelling didn't go away, but it didn't seem to get any worse either. When I got back home to my usual regimen, most of the swelling disappeared, but there was still a fullness in my upper arm."

Anita explained that her desire to limit problems before they grew huge motivated her to stick to a treatment plan, though it was challenging. "I didn't realize at first that I would need to wrap my arm both day and night," she said. "I struggled with my appearance, how the wrapping made me look like I'd had a major accident. It attracted immediate attention. I finally learned to tell people who asked that the bandages were for protection." She laughed. "It's funny, but nobody ever asked me what *kind* of protection. I don't know what I would have said if they had."

Wrapping presented a real dilemma when it came to fitting into her clothes. She said, "The bandages were so bulky, getting a long sleeve over them was impossible. I was wondering if I'd have to grapple with bandages for the rest of my life." She began wearing a compression sleeve during the day, though she still wrapped the arm in bandages most nights. Before she got the sleeve, she said, "The bandages would begin to itch and feel tight after about three or four hours, and I would look for things to distract myself with. The main distraction was eating. Then I started gaining weight and decided I was going to have a real problem if I didn't watch out." She found that the compression sleeve allowed a lot more freedom of movement and fit better under her clothes. As she put it, "I forget that it's there." She measured her arm regularly so she could determine what caused the swelling to flare up. "I'm getting a little sense of what I can and can't do," she said.

Besides wrapping and wearing the sleeve, Anita was careful to use lotions that helped maintain the health of her skin, and she was faithful to an exercise regimen. She started exercising just a few weeks after surgery, when her husband put up a basketball hoop and they began shooting hoops together. "It seemed like a logical thing for arm exercise," she said, "though I have to admit, winter put a crimp in it." She attended both a low-impact aerobic-dance class and yoga several times a week. She said, "I've been incorporating lymphedema exercises into the yoga routines. It took me almost a year not to be sore after the yoga sessions, because I have some arthritis."

Anita admitted that her complete regimen took a lot of effort. She said, "When I realized it was going to take such a chunk of time—an hour and a half or so every day—to massage and exercise and bandage, I first tried to just squeeze it in without changing anything in my daily schedule. It didn't work. I had to allow time for it, to make it a real commitment. Sometimes I get discouraged when I consider that I'm going to have to do some version of this for the rest of my life. It's like one more cost of having had breast cancer. But you can't let yourself lapse into self-defeating behaviors. Keeping my arm from ballooning is still important to me. I have the tools to deal with my lymphedema. I didn't have those before."

In a follow-up conversation five years after our first talk, Anita told me she was no longer bothered by lymphedema. "My lymphedema is really minimal now," she said. "I still watch my health. I go to yoga regularly and I think that might have improved the strength in my muscles. It's been a help." She added that she does not wrap or wear a sleeve unless she's gardening or flying. If she fails to do so, she does get some swelling. She said, "I was standing in line at the airport not long ago and saw another woman wearing a sleeve. I spoke to her, showed her my own sleeve, and we commiserated a moment before moving on." In the same way, Anita has moved on with her life.

18

SEEKING TREATMENT

When you or your doctor decides it is time to treat your lymphedema, you'll face many issues not only in the search for treatment but also in getting it paid for. In this chapter we make some suggestions about obtaining treatment and about securing insurance coverage for it. We also discuss legislative issues surrounding the coverage of treatments by insurance companies.

The good news is that the last several years have witnessed a great increase in the number of therapists throughout the United States who are trained to provide lymphedema care. It is most likely that your medical oncologist or radiation oncologist will have one or more qualified therapists with whom they work closely. Asking your doctor is a good way to begin looking for a lymphedema therapist. In addition, all the lymphedema training programs listed in the Resources section at the back of the book maintain lists of therapists who have been certified through their programs. You can find therapists organized by state or region on the websites of most training programs. You can also contact the programs by phone. Or you can contact your local hospital and ask questions similar to those listed below.

Questions to Ask when Considering a Treatment Program

Here is a list of questions you can use as a guideline when you are deciding on treatment. They are based on those suggested by the National Lymphedema Network.[1] Be sure to get all your own questions answered as well. Don't be embarrassed to question potential therapists about the treatment program they follow and about their background and training.

The Program

* What kinds of programs do you offer? Do they include manual lymphatic drainage or something comparable? Do they include myofascial release treatment?

* Would you use continuous compression during or after my therapy? If so, what kind (bandages, garments, etc.)?

* How long is your program? If I need longer treatment, would you provide it?

* Do I need authorization from my doctor to begin treatment?

* How much training do your therapists have? (In the United States and Europe the minimum training for certification is 135 to 150 hours.) Are the recommended therapists certified, either through individual training programs or with LANA (Lymphology Association of North America)?

* What results can I expect?

* Can I contact and get a recommendation from someone who has been through your program?

Products

* Do you sell bandages and compression garments, or do you have recommendations for where I can buy them?

* Are you qualified to measure me for garments, or is the supplier you recommend qualified to do the measurements?

Care after Treatment

* Will you train me to manage my lymphedema after treatment? Will you educate me in areas such as self-massage,

skin care, exercise regimens, diet, and complementary holistic therapies?

❋ Do you have a lymphedema support group, or do you know of one in the area?

❋ Do you provide emergency assistance, or help on holidays, weekends, and evenings?

Costs

❋ How much does the program cost?

❋ When will I pay for treatment?

❋ Can you bill my insurance company? If so, do I need a preauthorization before I begin treatment?

❋ Is there a cost for follow-up treatment?

Insurance

The last four or five years have brought some progress in the matter of insurance coverage for treatment of lymphedema. Nonetheless, not all carriers provide coverage for the condition, and when they do it can have gaps. Insurance coverage is worth checking into, because a single session of lymphedema treatment through a licensed practitioner will cost well over two hundred dollars.

Some private insurance companies still don't cover lymphedema at all. The only way to know if you're covered is to check with your provider. Most policies cover lymphedema in a piecemeal manner—some cover therapy, some cover the cost of supplies, some cover garments and bandages—but not many cover it all.

No matter what coverage you have, be sure to find out if treatment must be preauthorized by your carrier *before* you begin it. Some insurance carriers and HMOs only pay for care given by a practitioner who is listed in their plans as a preferred provider (or is directly employed by a preferred provider). If your insurance carrier does not have lists of approved therapists trained or certified in decongestive lymphatic therapy, request a referral to a practitioner outside the system. All insurance carriers have some kind of mechanism for covering outside services.

If your carrier says your plan doesn't cover lymphedema, work with your doctor or physical therapist to appeal the decision. Your doctor may be willing to write a letter to the insurance company detailing the medical necessity for lymphedema treatment. If even after an appeal your insurance company refuses coverage, you may still want to push for it. If you do, be prepared to provide the company with documentation about the effectiveness of treatment and the consequences of leaving your lymphedema untreated. Copy articles from the National Lymphedema Network's newsletter. Go to your library and find journals that support your stance. Show them this book.

Involve your doctor. She or he may have suggestions and strategies that can help get your insurance company to cover treatment. Phrases such as "manual lymph drainage," "lymphatic mobilization," "bandaging," and "exercise" are usually more acceptable to insurance companies than "massage," which is less likely to be covered.

Involve your therapist. Sometimes the lines between lymphedema and other conditions are blurred. If lymphedema is not the only condition for which you need treatment, perhaps your therapist can treat your lymphedema along with your other condition, which may be covered under your policy.

Point out the high costs that may be incurred by the insurance company from possible complications if your lymphedema is left untreated. Mention the potential for infections, skin disorders, and even hospitalization. Treatment for a single infection could equal the cost of lymphedema treatment. Document the status of your health regarding lymphedema; detail your functional limitations, your impairments, your goals. Itemize the treatment you need in order to improve your health.

Be sure to document all contact with your insurance carrier. Each time you speak with them, note the name of the person you spoke with and the date and time you talked. Keep copies of all letters you send plus copies of any information you include.

And don't forget to involve suppliers of lymphedema products. Most of them will be willing to work with you to get coverage. Adam Anschel, an employee of LymphaCare, a supplier of products used in treating lymphedema, works with lymphedema patients all the time. He says, "In most cases we are able to accept what the insurance allows, resulting in little to no out-of-pocket expense for our patients. We have had excellent success getting lymphedema products approved and reimbursed by Aetna, Blue Cross/Blue Shield, United-Healthcare, Cigna, Oxford, Humana, and many more."

Legislative Issues

Gradual progress has been made toward the enactment of laws that would require insurance carriers to provide coverage for lymphedema treatment. In April 1997 Senator Edward Kennedy (D-Mass.) introduced bill S-609, which passed in the Senate and was referred to the House of Representatives, where it was read twice and referred to the Committee on Labor and Human Resources. There has been no more action on it since then. If it were to pass, the bill would require that group and individual health plans provide coverage for reconstructive breast surgery if they provide coverage for mastectomies. They would also be mandated to cover the costs of complications from mastectomy, including lymphedema.

In 1998, President Clinton signed Public Law 105-277, the Women's Health and Cancer Rights Act. The law requires that, depending on individual policies' copayments, deductables, etc., they must provide coverage for mastectomies and related services, including all stages of reconstructive surgery; surgery and reconstruction to produce a symmetrical appearance; prostheses; and the treatment of physical complications, *including lymphedema*.

Another encouraging move has occurred in the area of Medicare coverage. In December 2003 the cap for physical and occupational therapies was lifted, but *only through December 31, 2005.* Unless pending legislation called the Medicare Access to Rehabilitation Services Act of 2005 (S-438/HR-916) is passed, which would keep the caps off rehabilitation therapy, the caps will be reinstated in 2006. The Medicare Access to Rehabilitation Services Act was introduced in the Senate in March 2003 by John Ensign (R-Nev.) and reads, in part, "To amend Title XVIII of the Social Security Act to repeal the Medicare outpatient rehabilitation therapy caps." The bill was supported by more than fifty senators, but it remains unpassed as of this writing.

Another important Medicare policy that impacts lymphedema patients went into effect in May 2005. The policy document states that only licensed physical therapists, physical therapist assistants, occupational therapists, occupational therapist assistants, and in some special instances nurse practitioners will be reimbursed for lymphedema treatments using rehabilitation billing codes to bill for CDT (complete decongestive therapy). This essentially prevents a number of experienced lymphedema practitioners, such as massage therapists and nurses, from obtaining Medicare reimbursement and may limit a lymphedema patient's ability to receive effective treatment.

The National Lymphedema Network encourages lymphedema patients and other concerned individuals to contact their congressional representatives and urge them to vote for passage of bill S-438/HR-916 and to ask them to amend the May 2005 policy that limits reimbursement for lymphedema treatment. The NLN website (www.lymphnet.org/caps.html) provides sample letters as well as information on how to reach your congressional representatives.

Until the seriousness of lymphedema is recognized and the need for up-to-date treatment is accepted by the medical community and by insurance providers, you will need to act as your own advocate. Write your representatives in Congress. Educate your doctor. Educate your insurance carrier. Form or join a support group with others who are grappling with the condition. Who knows? Maybe your efforts will be just the thing to push the system into action and get patients the help they need.

Next, Part Three of the book, "Beyond Conventional Treatments," takes a look at the emotional aspects of living with lymphedema, the powers of the mind and spirit to help heal the body, and complementary approaches to treatment.

part three

BEYOND
CONVENTIONAL
TREATMENTS

19

LYMPHEDEMA and EMOTIONS

The emotional discomfort brought on by lymphedema can be as fierce as the physical. For some patients, it's worse. The prospect of living with lymphedema can be scary, sad, and more than a little maddening. Medical oncologist Stephen Chandler says the majority of his patients who are affected by the condition become quite upset. "Fear, the heaviness of their arm, the feeling that nothing can be done—all these cause a great deal of apprehension," he says. "Many women panic, or they just make themselves put up with it, or they hide it until somebody tells them how to get help. Some of my elderly women patients have had lymphedema for years and do not know that there is help available to them now."

Even with increasing awareness and understanding of lymphedema, the medical community still tends to downplay or ignore its emotional component. However, for decades psychologists and therapists have been counseling patients suffering from the condition. Three therapists, Ruth Bach, M.Ed., L.P.C., Izetta Smith, M.A., and Vicki Romm, L.C.S.W., generously share their experience and insight in this chapter.

Therapists' Perspectives

Ruth Bach, who has been a therapist for more than twenty years, heads the cancer counseling center at a large medical facility. She gives us the benefit of her experience not only as a therapist but also, in the next chapter, as a patient. "Having lymphedema can be real depressing," she says. "And for so many years, women were told they just had to live with their lymphedema. They often became depressed, and then they found no help for their depression." A study conducted in London in the early 1990s confirms Ruth's statement.[1] Of the one hundred women who participated in the study—all of them breast cancer patients—half had resulting arm swelling and the other half did not. The women with swelling had experienced it for an average of about fifty months. All the participants were assessed as to both functional and psychiatric ability or impairment. The study reported, "Patients with arm swelling... experienced functional impairment, psychosocial maladjustment, and increased psychological morbidity." They also experienced difficulty in their home environments and in familial relationships. The women who had no arm swelling appeared better able to assimilate the whole experience of breast cancer and to put it behind them and get on with their lives.

Ruth says that although health-care professionals still must educate people about lymphedema, she's noticed an emerging openness about it. "There's more permission to talk about it than there used to be. It's validating to patients to acknowledge the importance of the quality of life. In the past it was like pulling teeth to get doctors to advise women to see a psychologist. And when women did, they felt such relief.... A huge part of our job as counselors is to allow women to realize it is normal to feel the way they do. A woman feels validation when a counselor acknowledges to her that it is okay to pay attention to what she is feeling."

Family and friends don't seem to understand the emotional downside of lymphedema. For loved ones of cancer survivors, Ruth says, "Lymphedema seems too far down the line" of what is important. "The cancer diagnosis is so urgent, nothing else really matters. People close to cancer patients seem to relay a message that says, 'You're okay without breasts, you're okay with all the changes in you. We're just glad you're here.' " Therapists, she says, "can provide women with the knowledge that they are not alone, that they are not weird, that they or their bodies have not done something wrong to cause the cancer or the lymphedema. And we show them there are solutions, even if they have to search to find those solutions. Then, when many of the women see the results of physical therapy, they are thrilled. Most of them keep up with the program, wrapping and doing exercises."

Still, Ruth adds, no matter how successful treatment is, no matter how much peace of mind women achieve about their condition, misgivings may linger. She says, "When women realize this is ongoing and that they will be dealing with it the rest of their lives, they are likely to have regrets. It's alright not to like that this happened to you, but there is hope you can at least gain some control over it and can feel normal again. Counseling can have a huge effect on learning how to get through all of what we need to get through."

Izetta Smith, who has counseled women with breast cancer and lymphedema for almost ten years, is emphatic about the effects of cancer and its treatment on women's emotions. "When women experience breast cancer," she says, "a range of different things can affect their day-to-day lives. There are those lucky women who don't experience many physical changes. But others undergo some real and immediate changes. Some women have almost instant menopause or perimenopause—with lowered libidos, hot flashes, and mood swings—because of the changes in estrogen [in their bodies]. There are also changes in their bodies after surgery. There is the need to deal with hair loss after chemotherapy. Normally, when we see a woman who is flooded with these events, it's all she can talk about, all she can think about."

Izetta says most women deal with the issues and manage to get on with living. "But," she says, "if a woman gets lymphedema a year or two after cancer, she finds another load to handle. With some women, it's almost as if this new problem stimulates the feelings of the original diagnosis of cancer, recycling the grief that came with the cancer. It can be a real, deep letdown. There are so many feelings of loss with cancer, big losses as well as little ones, some you may not feel until many years later. Cancer can truly bring a loss of innocence. Lymphedema can seem like another doorway into looking at what you have lost." In groups she facilitates for cancer survivors, women often say they feel lymphedema is a deformity. She says,

"They find they can't button their sleeves, they have to quit wearing their jewelry, they have to wear different clothes. And for some women, there is physical discomfort as well. Even if a woman does not have issues about her body image, even if the swelling is not important to her, she may have to deal with pain."

Vicki Romm, who has been a practicing therapist for twenty years, concurs. She says. "As women go along, they pass through the stages of treatment and healing and they begin to think they're done, and normally they come to a place of being okay with the breast cancer. Then the lymphedema is dumped on them. It can have as much of an effect on their emotions as the initial diagnosis of cancer. They have to revisit emotions they came to believe they'd moved beyond." One such feeling is fear. "It's not unusual for someone to feel incredible fear about what lymphedema is and what it might mean," Vicki says. "We need to help women 'normalize' the lymphedema, to make them realize it is not unique to them."

Izetta Smith adds, "I think if women learned after surgery that there was the possibility of lymphedema, they would take more care in trying to prevent it. It's sad that we had no resources [for educating cancer patients about lymphedema and its treatment] until recently. When women came to us with lymphedema, we had nowhere to send them. Now we do." At the same time, she says, "We still take the same care with them as we ever did. We try to draw them out, to help them get to a place where they can deal with the emotional issues—and believe me, there are some deep emotional issues with it."

Vicki and Izetta agree that their task is to encourage women to talk about the feelings connected with lymphedema—to explore not only its physical but also its emotional effects. Still, as concerned as they are with their patients' emotional well-being, they are also acutely aware of patients' need for more information on all aspects of treatment, and the earlier the better. Recent advances in the treatment and prevention of lymphedema indicate that education is extremely important.[2] Vicki believes that everyone who is treated for breast cancer should be sent to a lymphedema clinic. "As I've learned more about lymphedema," she says, "it occurs to me that women should be sent to physical therapy or to some kind of class to learn about lymphedema even *before* lymph node dissection."

Izetta says, "We have to encourage them to demand help from their doctors. They must insist on seeing someone who is trained and experienced in the specific treatments for lymphedema—not just someone who does normal massage, but someone who knows how to do lymphatic massage.... A woman must not take no for an answer. There is treatment available even if her doctor doesn't know about it. She needs to insist that she get it. She is her own best advocate."

Help for Dealing with Difficult Emotions

Where can you find help for exploring the many feelings that may crop up as you adjust to living with lymphedema? A good place to start is through your health-care provider. Ask your doctor for a referral to a good therapist. Most patients have access to counseling services through their health coverage. The counseling coverage may not be *specifically* for lymphedema, but professional therapists can help their clients deal with issues related to whatever is throwing a wrench into their emotional lives, whether it be physical health, depression, family issues, or substance abuse.

Another idea is to find a support group for people with lymphedema. You may be lucky enough that your health-care provider actually sponsors a group for lymphedema patients. But many do not. If that's the case, yours may know where to send you to find one. If they can't, the National Lymphedema Network maintains a list of lymphedema support groups, including their locations, phone numbers, and meeting dates. Call the NLN (see Resources) or check its website at www.lymphnet.org/support. If you are unable to locate a group in your community, consider starting one yourself. Again, the National Lymphedema Network provides great information on organizing a support group; check www.lymphnet.org/setupsupport.

If you have Internet access, you can connect with the online lymphedema community. A wonderful source of support is the website operated by Lymphedema People (www.lymphedemapeople

.com). There you'll find information about most aspects of the illness and its treatment, links to chatrooms and online discussions, answers to questions—a whole array of assistance. There's a complete section in Spanish, too.

It might take some work and time to reach it, but emotional balance can be within your grasp again. In Chapter 21, "The Powers of Mind and Spirit," you'll learn even more ways to go about taking your life back. It is worth the effort to jettison any emotional baggage you might be carrying and to replace it with things that nurture and ground your mind, heart, and spirit. As Jean emphasized in her comments about working with lymphedema patients (Chapter 4), those who were proactive in figuring out how to get on with their lives—"those who get out and live life, who walk, swim, ride bikes," as she put it—were the ones who fared the best.

So, friend, if you find yourself in the grip of emotional turmoil, first of all, realize you're not alone. Reach out. Connect with the thousands of others who can help you get through it. Then, once you've reestablished your footing, reach out and help others reclaim their emotional health. Life can go on, and even for those with lymphedema it can be plenty nice when it does.

20

RUTH'S STORY
a COUNSELOR TREATS HERSELF
and OTHERS

Ruth Bach, whom we met in the last chapter, counsels cancer patients and manages a counseling center that treats dozens of cancer patients and their families each month. She is trim and fashionable, wearing an almost ankle-length skirt and black tunic. Her observations about the effects of cancer and lymphedema on emotional health come from the almost three decades she's spent as a therapist as well as from her own experiences as a patient. "I think," she says, "that depression is a response to the unendingness of things. In our society we're geared for flight or fight. Depression can take the form of flight. We depress ourselves so we don't feel the anxiety. Depression can help dull the sharpness of our pain. We are geared for resolution, and lymphedema is hard to resolve."

Ruth had been counseling women with breast cancer for seven years when she herself was diagnosed with it. She had a lumpectomy, and her lymph nodes were removed for staging. "Knowing other women with breast cancer really helped me deal with my own cancer," she says. "I don't think I needed to have breast cancer to be a good counselor, but I feel it deepened my understanding—although I am also aware we are all individuals, that no two of us are alike. In each of us there are pockets, secret places, that no one will ever know or understand."

She continues, "One of the greatest aids to survival is having a sense of meaning and a sense that you belong to a community, a place where you have a connection. Health and recovery depend on it." Her words come fast, as if she is eager to help every woman. "We have to speak up about our problems. We can't simply go on and"— she fingers quote marks in the air—" 'live with it' alone. It used to be the case with cancer. We were told we just had to live with it. It's now typical with lymphedema. Yes, you have to live with it, but that doesn't mean do nothing about it. Don't accept the 'There's nothing we can do' answer. If we are told there is nothing to be done, we need to ask, 'Then *who* can help me?' If you are not getting help or your questions aren't answered by your doctor, go to your cancer counselor, go to other cancer patients, call the advice nurses, talk to a physical therapist. There is help, but sometimes you need to search to find it."

Six years after Ruth's first bout with cancer she had a recurrence, which was treated with a mastectomy and chemotherapy. She remembers precisely when she developed lymphedema. "It had been six years since the nodes were removed," she says. "For six years I had no problems at all. Then, not long after the second surgery, I was gardening, cutting up little limbs from a tree we had trimmed. Two days later," she holds out her right arm, which is slim and elegant, "my arm just ballooned. I think I was more upset with the swelling than I was at any time with the cancer. I was working in the medical community at that time, but no one knew about massage for swelling, or bandaging, or any of the techniques that are coming along now."

On her own she found a compression sleeve, which she wore twenty-four hours a day for a year. Finally the swelling went away, except for "one little bump" just above the elbow. "I keep working at it," she says. "And I do this little mini-exercise." She shows how she pushes her fingers up her arm, toward her shoulder.

She says, "It is normal and healthy to be obsessive when something is wrong with you, particularly in the beginning. Sometimes obsession is our way of moving on. And it is healthy if in the process it helps you get through. Sometimes we *need* to focus, to obsess. I think often we push things away in our society. So pushing away, making the best of it, becomes our normal response. But in order to take care of your body, you *have* to think about it. I think it's important to pay attention, in order to give yourself quality. Nothing matters without that. Self-esteem and ego are really important."

She holds out her arm again and tenderly strokes it. "For all practical purposes my lymphedema is gone. I use the tendons as my sign of whether it's swollen or not. I really watch to make sure I can still see them." She wears a compression sleeve if she is going to do heavy work, or iron. She laughs, "Even with fabrics like they are today, I still like to iron now and then." She adds that she works out with barbells every morning, without fail, and works with stationary weights and free weights three times a week. She says, "If I don't do it everyday I get little creaks and tingles." Still, she wakes up some mornings with a sensation that makes her worry. "My arm will feel tired, or heavy, or like something is going on. I don't know if it's in my imagination or not, but I don't like it. Sometimes I would love to take a vacation from the exercise drill." She laughs. "*Everybody* takes vacations. But I really can't. If I want to keep the swelling down, it's just something I am going to have to do forever."

As we conclude she says, "It occurs to me there are improvements in [cancer] diagnosis that spare the lymph nodes in some women. And that is going to pose a dilemma for us who came before. I see that same dilemma in women who had the old-fashioned radical mastectomy." Her face grows stern. "Talk about deformity! Talk about immobility! I've had to counsel them and deal with their rage and their sorrow when they begin thinking they had cancer too early. We are going to experience that sorrow and regret ourselves one day. There *are* going to be improvements. Women in the future will not have to suffer as much as we do. And we must recognize and express our feelings about that. There has to be room for the protest. We have to let the two-year-old in us stamp her foot and scream. It doesn't make the pain go away, but it lets us honor ourselves and our experiences. We have to have room to say it."

21

the POWERS *of* MIND *and* SPIRIT

From a holistic point of view, health and wellness include mental health and spiritual contentment as well as physical health and emotional well-being. In this chapter we look at the effects of stress on our lives and the potential benefits of relaxation, meditation, prayer, and visualization for people with lymphedema.

Medical oncologist Stephen Chandler has seen positive effects in some of his patients who have incorporated nontraditional practices into their health regimes alongside regular medical treatments. "In my practice," he says, "I'm encouraging people to strengthen their emotional, spiritual, and immune systems all together, to take everything into account: massage, walking, acupuncture, prayer. The benefits of all these things are becoming scientifically proven." He laughs and says, "Only in our country would we try to scientifically prove the effects of prayer. But some PET scans show improvement after prayer." (PET is short for *positron emission tomography*; a PET scan is an X ray that can show hot spots of activity in the body, which are commonly areas of cancer activity where there is rapid cell division.) He continues, "Our whole body does not respond well when we aren't taking care of ourselves, like when we don't eat right or get enough rest or sleep."

As Dr. Chandler says, it is our "whole" self that gives us health— indeed, both *whole* and *health* come from the same root word—and finding wholeness is the subject of this chapter. You may already be using some of the ideas presented here. If so, good for you. If not, consider doing so. Not only can they enhance healing, but they can also make life fuller.

The Power of the Mind to Heal

Perhaps some of our most potent strengths lie in the power of our minds. As related in his book *Anatomy of an Illness*, Norman Cousins had a disease that was destroying the connective tissues in his spine and joints.[1] Sick and in the hospital, Cousins began to think that illness could come from a person's thoughts as much as it could from accident, trauma, disease, or genetics. He hypothesized that the reverse may also be true: If he could heal his own mind, his body would follow. He asked for some old Marx brothers' movies and film clips from *Candid Camera* to be sent to his room. And when he watched them, he started laughing. The results were almost immediate. Ten minutes of belly laughs gave him two hours of pain-free sleep without the benefit of any other painkillers. Even more important, the results were cumulative. After each session of laughter, his health continued to improve. He writes, "I have learned never to underestimate the capacity of the human mind and body to regenerate."[2]

The powerful benefit of laughter and humor in Norman Cousins' case is not an isolated event. The benefits of laughter are well documented and have been scientifically studied.[3,4,5] Laughter exercises the lungs and the circulatory system, increases the amount of oxygen in the blood, and boosts the immune system. "He who laughs, lasts!" says author Mary Pettibone Poole. The specific link between laughter and the treatment and management of lymphedema is not yet documented, but we know at a minimum that laughter stimulates diaphragmatic breathing, which helps boost lymph flow. And why not have a little fun trying it?

The Effects of Stress

One way we can harness the power of the mind to heal is by becoming aware of how we handle stress. Our lives are filled with stress, and when we experience it our bodies respond instantly: our muscles tense, our system releases adrenaline, our metabolism speeds up, we breathe faster, our blood-sugar level rises, our heart speeds up, our blood pressure increases, and our blood supply is diverted from the stomach to the extremities. In other words, our body prepares us to fight or to flee.

When we experience it in short bursts, stress serves an important purpose: It prepares us to respond to danger. But if stress becomes chronic, it can lower the body's immune response and can weaken—even damage—our systems. No one lives without stress, so knowing how to deal with it is an important ingredient in health. All of us have come down with a cold or the flu when we were under a great deal of stress. In fact, some cancer patients say they felt the cancer coming on during a particularly stressful time. Certain life events greatly heighten stress levels. Here is a short list of the most potent of them:[6]

* Death of a spouse

* Divorce

* Marital separation

* Serving a jail term

* Death of a close family member

* Personal injury or illness

* Marriage

* Being fired from a job

* Marital reconciliation

* Retirement

* Change in the health of a family member

* Pregnancy

* Sexual difficulties

* Gaining a new family member

* Business readjustment

...and the list goes on.

Since you can't control all external events, your mission is to take charge of how you respond to them. Half the battle is realizing when stress has you in its grip. Be aware of times when your shoulders are pulling up toward your ears, your chest is tightening, you're clenching your teeth, or you're holding your breath or breathing faster. Picture this: You're stuck in heavy traffic, and as a result you're late for a job interview for which you spent three days rewriting your resume. You are stopped dead at an intersection. Every time the light changes from green to yellow to red your neck muscles cramp. Your fingers clutch the wheel and blanch. You grit your teeth and hold your breath. You are growing both angry and scared that you'll miss out on the perfect job—the *only* job you'll ever have again in your life. You're a mess.

Will the tension you're storing up make the traffic move? Will you get to the interview any faster by holding your breath? And how will you perform if you arrive feeling like you do? Why not, right there in the middle of the tailpipe exhaust, make a change? Why not unknot your stomach and give yourself a break? Do this: Let your hands relax in your lap. Drop your shoulders and begin to breathe. Practice what you learned in the chapter on belly breathing. Slowly inhale through your nose, and allow the breath to go deep, moving only your stomach. Whisper the breath out through your lips. Keep breathing steadily and rhythmically. Concentrate on letting go, on how you feel; literally picture the cramped muscles in your neck unknotting.

You have a choice. You can make yourself feel better. You will eventually get to the interview. How you feel when you get there is up to you.

The Benefits of Relaxation

Feeling better is the best outcome of relaxing, and it is the product of many physiological changes. When we relax, our systems do an about-face. Our blood pressure drops, our breathing slows, our muscles relax, and our metabolic rate decreases. Bottom line: Being relaxed is a healthful state. However, unlike the stress response, which can be triggered unconsciously, relaxation takes a conscious effort to achieve.[7] With practice, a relaxation response can be triggered immediately, perhaps with diaphragmatic breathing as the cue.

The list of tools that can help manage stress is long. To discover what works best for us, we need to experiment. Some well-known options include:

* Engaging in regular exercise

* Practicing good nutrition

* Getting adequate sleep

* Minimizing emotional stressors (noisy environments, bright colors, extreme temperatures, strong smells, clutter, etc.)

* Surrounding yourself with people who support you (rather than drain you)

* Practicing belly breathing and pursuing progressive relaxation techniques

Dr. Herbert Benson, head of the Mind/Body Medical Institute at Harvard Medical School and author of the book *The Relaxation Response*, has studied the physiological effects of meditation, relaxation, and prayer for several years. An article in the *New York Times* quotes him as saying, "There are many activities you can use to evoke the relaxation response: yoga, meditation, running, music." He adds that about 80 percent of his patients choose prayer.[8] In other interviews Benson says relaxation requires two basic steps: The first is to stop thinking of everyday troubles. "One of the most effective ways to do this is through repetition: repeating a word, a sound, a thought, a breathing exercise or even a religious phrase."[7] He gives examples: "Christians might use 'Our Father who art in heaven,' Jews might choose 'Shalom,' a Hindu might use 'Om.'" He says that words like *peace, calm,* or *ocean* can work as well.[9] The second step is to take time to relax *every day*—in fact, twice a day is best—for ten to twenty minutes. It can take a month to perfect the practice, but soon your body will automatically respond to stress with much less ferocity than it once did.

Meditation and Visualization

We have known for a long time that a mind-body connection exists, but it remains little understood and difficult to document. Carl and Stephanie Simonton, working with cancer patients in the early 1970s, used techniques of imagery and visualization to promote healing. Surgeon Bernie Siegel, author of *Love, Medicine, and Miracles*, a book about the psychology of healing, expanded upon their work. He observed that in cancer patients healing occurred in response to techniques of relaxation, meditation, hypnosis, and visualization.[10] In 2002 Gregg D. Jacobs, an assistant professor of psychiatry at Harvard Medical School, wrote in the *Journal of Alternative Complementary Medicine* that mind-body interactions are real and can be measured.[11] This section examines two mental practices that are often credited with promoting a healing effect in the body: meditation and visualization.

In her book *Minding the Body, Mending the Mind*, Joan Borysenko defines meditation as "any activity that keeps the attention pleasantly anchored in the present moment."[12] Bernie Siegel describes it is a method by which one can "temporarily stop listening to the pressures and distractions of everyday life" and become more aligned with one's "deeper thoughts and feelings, the peace of pure consciousness, and spiritual awareness."[13] The initial focus of many forms of meditation is breathing—simply noticing the breath as it flows in and out. Some teachers recommend repeating phrases or sounds that are meaningful to you, for example, "peace," "love," "nice and easy," or "let go," or sounds such as "mmmm" or "nnnn." Sometimes picturing a single relaxing image, such as that of a candle flame, works well. It is important for you to pick your own words, sounds, or images, choosing those that free your mind from its accustomed busy-ness and allow you to focus on *just being*.

As simple as it sounds, this settling in and finding internal serenity can be challenging because our culture doesn't strongly embrace internal serenity; rather, it pressures us to act and rewards us for keeping busy. Many of us find it hard to allow ourselves even short periods of inactivity and quiet. But hanging in there and developing a regular meditation practice is worth it. People who consistently meditate enjoy improved concentration and, eventually, a sense of calmness that helps them to deal better with life's daily challenges. The stress response is minimized, leading to greater emotional, mental, and physical well-being. Bernie Siegel writes, "I know of no other single activity that by itself can produce such great improvement in the quality of life."[14]

Visualization, a practice combining relaxation or meditation techniques with specific mental imagery, taps into a curious phenomenon: The human body cannot distinguish between a vivid mental experience and an actual physical one. Much clinical evidence supports the theory that visualization can produce a powerful physical response. Electromyography, the study of electrical activity in muscle, has shown that simply imagining an activity electrically activates the muscles that are used to perform the activity.

Guidelines for visualization suggest that you choose an image to focus on that is realistic, believable for you, and can be seen clearly in the mind's eye. Bernie Siegel notes that the Simontons made an initial misjudgment by speculating that all patients would respond to an image involving fighting and warfare to kill their cancer cells. But many people were disturbed by such images and as a result had difficulty relaxing when they used them. A more helpful visualization might be one in which an army of white blood cells carries the cancer cells away. Dr. Siegel tells of a child who visualized his cancer as cat food and the immune cells as white cats.[15]

For someone with lymphedema, suggestions for visualizations might include the following:

* See the existing, healthy lymph vessels expanding, allowing lymph to flow out of the arm.

* Visualize little rivers of lymph flowing into new channels up and over the top of your shoulder, or across the midline of your body to a new quadrant.

* Visualize alternative pathways of flow that detour around the impaired lymph system.

* Visualize the lymph nodes throughout your body pumping effectively (in much the same way you can imagine the heart pumping).

* Visualize each lymph angion (the individual segment of lymph vessel) pumping fluid forward to the next angion, and that one pumping to the next, and so on.

* Focus on the lymph vessels' one-way valves opening and then closing to prevent the backflow of lymph fluid.

* Focus on your diaphragmatic breathing, and visualize the pressure changes in the thoracic cavity gently stimulating the large lymphatic vessels in the trunk.

* See yourself with a smaller limb, and perhaps wearing clothes to show it off.

* As you exercise while wearing a compression bandage, visualize the lymph vessels being gently squeezed between the muscle and the bandaged skin, moving lymph fluid up your arm.

* During lymphatic massage, visualize it assisting the flow of fluid.

Use your imagination to create other visualizations that have meaning for you. The choices are limitless.

Here are some more tips for enhancing your visualization practice: Modify your aural environment by surrounding yourself with sounds that calm you and help you focus: soft music, nature sounds, "white" noise. Some people find it helpful to make an audiotape of a "script" to guide their visualizations. (Below, we have provided an example of one.) Others prefer to guide the images mentally. To be most effective, visualization is best practiced regularly over a period of several weeks. It is not realistic to do it once and expect significant results.

We can only scratch the surface of the topic here. Many publications, audiotapes, and videotapes are available that offer background information on visualization and guidelines for developing a practice. Hundreds of practitioners are trained in visualization techniques, and some of them lead classes. Ask a cancer counselor or any professional therapist if they can recommend good resources for learning more about visualization for medical conditions.

A Suggested Visualization

Place yourself in a comfortable position, preferably sitting with your hands and feet uncrossed. Become aware of your breathing and the motion of your chest and abdomen. Slowly breathe in and out, noticing the gentle flow of air. Breathe in peace and breathe out tension. Close your eyes if doing so is comfortable for you. Starting at your forehead and working downward to your toes, focus on each area of the body one at a time. You may want to physically tighten and release the muscles in each successive area. Notice the gradual release of tension as you move your awareness through your body. Your body may begin to feel heavy or warm.

Picture a pleasant scene, one that is a safe place for you. Imagine the colors, aromas, and sounds. This is your corner of the universe, a place where wellness exists. Find somewhere to sit down in your scene. Take a few moments to just be there, allowing the warmth of the sun and the energy of the earth to heal you. Here, you are safe and at peace.

Next, move your awareness to the area of your body that is swollen with lymphedema. Visualize the lymph fluid leaving the area, and picture it flowing to new areas that can take care of it. Add whatever images—perhaps including some from the above list—you think would be helpful.

After spending several minutes with the images you have chosen, let your awareness return to your entire body, perhaps noting the position you are in, the pressure of the chair against your back, the motion of your chest and abdomen as you breathe. Gradually bring your focus and attention back to the room.

To conclude the session take several slow, deep, cleansing breaths, becoming more alert and awake with each one. Allow yourself some quiet time to feel the benefits of the session before returning to your regular routine.

Dr. Chandler says, "It is so important for all of us to discard that which clutters our lives. The media in this country seem obsessed by things that have little meaning. I feel that women must let go of some of the loads in their lives." He continues, "Athletes aim to be in what they call the 'zone,' where outside and inside are absolutely one. The body is a healing machine, but you must let go sometimes as well. If everything is not perfect, if your edema continues, you are not a failure. You do the most you can, then you move on down the river."

Each of us is unique. Each of us finds peace and comfort in her own creative way. Now is the time to discover and embrace every lovely thing that nurtures your spirit: the cinnamon candle, the lavendar sachet, the droplets of sandalwood oil in your bath, the room filled with Mendelssohn or sitar music or the songs of Jimmy Buffett. However we do it, if we go quiet inside and listen to the whispers of our hearts, we can be filled with health, peace, and power.

22

FEATHER'S STORY
a CREATIVE APPROACH to HEALING

When we first met, Feather had been a psychiatric nurse for almost fifteen years. She had finished her studies late in life, after her children were grown. Her Eastern-themed clothes were dramatic and hip. She wore a cotton tunic and loose, drapey slacks with an ornate Indian paisley design. Green earrings dangled from her ears. Round-faced and blue-eyed, she was in her sixties, but her youthful features belied her age.

She said, "I was diagnosed with cancer three years ago, and I decided at the time I wasn't going to let it get the better of me. I set my mind to getting rid of it. The doctors wanted to dwell on statistics. But I am not a statistic. The mind is the most powerful organ in the body. The doctors couldn't know what I could do." She had a mastectomy and reconstruction during the same operation. She had to convince the surgeon to do both procedures at once. Her hospital was not performing them together at the time, though she knew of others that were. She insisted that if the hospital did not do as she wanted she would find one that did.

She said, "I did so well and was feeling so good a couple of weeks after the surgery that I decided to redo the floor in my living room. I had no idea I needed to be careful about heavy, repetitive work, and after a couple of days my arm swelled way up." She became quite animated as she told her story. "I called my counselor in tears. I was just beginning to feel like I was living again and on the road to recovery. Then this swelling came on. The counselor didn't have any idea what to suggest. I searched everywhere for help. My oncologist didn't know what to tell me. For two years I had lymphedema. I was crying out for help and no one knew how to help me."

Eventually she heard about lymphedema massage. It wasn't available at her medical facility, and her insurance didn't cover it. She said, "I was beginning to think I was going to have to fight again to make them give me a referral to an outside practitioner. As it turned out, because I was so insistent, my medical facility sent someone to training. I was my therapist's first patient. And the swelling started to subside."

About a month prior to our meeting, Feather had undergone surgery to loosen some of the scar tissue remaining from the mastectomy. The surgical site became infected, and her arm swelled again. She showed me the arm, the lower part of which was larger than the other one. She said, "I don't feel so panicked this time. I know what to do about it. I am sporadic about bandaging. I do it maybe once a week. But I do qigong every morning and am finding that it helps." Feather learned qigong from Master Chen Hui-Xien, who herself had been diagnosed with a particularly virulent form of breast cancer fifteen years before. The doctors told Chen Hui-Xien she had three or four weeks to live. She refused to accept their prognosis and set out to search for a cure and to rehabilitate for herself. She discovered a form of qigong she called Soaring Crane.

"Qigong means life-breath, life-work, energy," Feather said. "Breathing oxygenates your body. Qigong is as ancient as tai chi. But it is not like tai chi, which is a martial art. Qigong is strictly for healing and health. It teaches breathing and visualizing to bring in the universal energy. You learn to exhale in ways that rid your body of the disease." She waved her arms gently over her head. "Like a soaring crane," she said.

Feather became very ill during chemotherapy. "But every morning," she said, "or almost every morning, I went to a special garden near a mansion in town. The garden was hidden behind a forest of trees. There, before anyone was up, I breathed and did qigong. I always came home feeling better. I think qigong is why my lymphedema is not too bad anymore, even after the infection."

She continued, "These last three years have been a gift for me, really. I feel an opportunity for aliveness. My connections with people are so much deeper. Everything has deepened—the spiritual, the reason to be alive. I have learned to be very, very kind—kind with my surgeons, with my therapist, with all the people working with me. I have compassion for them. I wanted them involved in my healing, and I feel these thoughts have helped everyone work better on me." She laughed. "Though I'll tell you, I wasn't going to let anybody cut on me who I didn't know."

She said, "I feel so blessed, so unafraid now. I have an opportunity to be on the path of gratitude. Once I decided I really wanted to live, it was like infinite connections came: new friends, fascinating learning, energy."

Five years later, Feather and I met again. She still was working as a nurse, and she was in the middle of redecorating her condo in an Oriental theme. She was studying Eastern calligraphy and practiced yoga and meditation. She had found a yoga teacher who specialized in working with what Feather called "older bodies." As for lymphedema, she had recently gone back to her therapist for six sessions of treatment, "to see what was new." Afterward, the swelling in her arm reduced even further than it had originally. The arm with lymphedema was now almost the same size as her other arm.

She said she wears a sleeve when she flies or gardens. She massages and does lymphedema exercises in the morning when she wakes up, and sometimes she puts Kiniesiotape along the top of her shoulder. "It's a chronic thing," she said, "but I don't make a big deal out of it. I don't focus on it. What you focus on becomes you. You have to appreciate what you have. I think all your life you have to tap into your aliveness."

23

COMPLEMENTARY THERAPIES
and
EMERGING TECHNOLOGIES

Quite a lot has changed in the world of lymphedema therapy in the last four or five years. We have learned more about the illness and we have expanded the possibilities for treatment. More and more people with lymphedema—indeed, with medical conditions of all kinds—are using alternative or complementary treatments. In fact doctors in Vermont report that over 70 percent of patients there use alternative therapies—and they are not shy about telling their doctors that they do.[1]

Though researchers have yet to discover a single pill that takes down the swelling of lymphedema or a one-stop method that puts everything right again, some exciting possibilities exist for complementary treatments. That is the topic of this chapter. It is important to realize that therapies like the ones described here are meant only to *complement* traditional treatments, not to replace them. And before you begin any new therapy, inform your doctor and other care practitioners about your plans to do so, in case you are taking any medications or receiving any treatments that could harmfully interact with it. Your good health depends on an educated health-care team.

Naturopathy and Acupuncture

Edythe Vickers, B.Sc., N.D., L.Ac., is a licensed acupuncturist and has been a practicing naturopathic physician for eighteen years. The clinic she directs specializes in acupuncture, naturopathic medicine, and holistic healing. Dr. Vickers has treated many patients with lymphedema. Typically, she gives them a referral to a lymphedema therapist, but she also interviews them and assesses their overall health and diet. She emphasizes the need to approach lymphedema the same way we should approach our health in general: as a whole. "I am concerned about what else is going on in their bodies," she says. "Do they smoke? Eat well? Exercise? What is their diet? If they're used to taking herbs, I may start with an herbal formula and lifestyle counseling, or if not I'll start with basic body balancing to reach their goals.... I look at balance, at the whole person, what they need, what they are willing to do."

Dr. Vickers stresses the importance of a healthy diet and educates patients about their bodies' essential water needs. Sufficient intake of water, she says, is imperative for good health. To determine the amount of water a person needs, she says, they should divide their body weight (in pounds) in half. The resulting number is how many ounces of water they should be drinking every day. Most people, she believes, do not drink nearly enough water. As for treating lymphedema, she says, "I want them to think about doing only one thing at a time." She recommends taking a few supplements daily, including calcium, magnesium, vitamin D, fish oil, and fiber (in the form of two to four tablespoons of flaxseed per day). She also prescribes green tea for its polyphenols, as well as milk thistle, Pycnogenols, and selenium. She recommends that all of her patients with cancer take Quercenol, a multiple-antioxidant pill. (A few of these supplements are described later in the chapter.)

Dr. Vickers has been successful using acupuncture needles directly on an area affected by lymphedema (and she says the practice is common in China), but many of her patients are aware of the precaution against using needles on an affected limb. She gives each patient a choice in whether or not to do acupuncture directly on the affected area. She is aware that one of the arguments against using acupuncture needles with lymphedema is the possibility of the introduction of bacteria into the affected tissue, but acupuncture needles are extremely small, sterile, and disposed of immediately after being used once. In addition, the sites on the skin are meticulously cleaned before treatment. Dr. Vickers maintains that the risk of infection under these conditions is infinitesimally small. "I've never seen a needle cause lymphedema," she says. She has also done acupuncture "with good results" on the arms and hands of doctors and other professionals whose lymphedema hinders their ability to practice. Sometimes she combines acupuncture with moxibustion, a treatment involving the herb mugwort, which when heated increases blood circulation. She says she has seen the combination of acupuncture and moxibustion immediately reduce lymphedema-related swelling. When a patient is treated with acupuncture, she says, "Lymphedema seems to stay away longer, unless the patient reaggravates it."

Dr. Vickers advises that anyone seeking naturopathic treatment or acupuncture should first ask the practitioner how much experience she or he has had working with cancer patients and with lymphedema. She recommends finding licensed practitioners through the American Association of Naturopathic Physicians (AANP) or the National Certification Commission for Acupuncture and Oriental Medicine (NCCAOM). See Resources.

Emerging Technologies

Therapies continue to be developed that take advantage of ongoing improvements in medical technology. One or more of them may be appropriate for you as an adjunct to conventional treatment for lymphedema.

Laser Treatment

A procedure using a sleeve-type mechanism that casts a low-level laser beam onto the patient's arm or torso is beginning to show promise in the treatment of lymphedema. Developed in Australia, the technique is thought to increase lymph viscosity (flow). In a study done at Flinders University, in Adelaide, no results showed up for one to three months after a series of two treatment cycles. But when the effects kicked in, the results were impressive. Nearly a third of the patients treated with the laser had a significant reduction in swelling and a softening of tissue in the affected arm, though they experienced no improvement in range of motion.[2]

Though using laser treatment for lymphedema is not currently standard practice in the United States, Vladimir Zharov, at the University of Arkansas for Medical Sciences, is working to develop the technology further, after having tested it in Russia in the late 1990s. More clinical testing is planned, and the method is under consideration by the U.S. Food and Drug Administration.

Infrared Therapy

Infrared therapy, another technology that uses light, is said to improve blood circulation and oxygenate tissue. It has been used for some time in the treatment of wounds that won't heal and is beginning to be looked at for treating lymphedema. So far no research on that application has been published in peer-reviewed journals, but practitioners are beginning to report results with some of their patients. We expect that, in the near future, clinical studies will be conducted on the effectiveness of this technology in treating lymphedema.

Hyperbaric Oxygenation

Hyperbaric oxygenation involves treating the entire body (not just the area affected by lymphedema) with 100 percent oxygen that has been pressurized to levels that are greater than normal. The process increases the concentration of oxygen in all the body's tissues and stimulates the growth of new blood vessels in areas with reduced circulation. It dilates the blood vessels, which again improves blood flow. It also stimulates the body's production of antioxidants and free-radical scavengers.

So, how can these effects treat lymphedema? That is what a research trial in England is trying to determine. A preliminary study showed some hopeful results. Three out of nineteen patients experienced more than 20 percent reduction in swelling after treatment, and six out of thirteen experienced more than 25 percent reduction. After twelve months, however, the reduction was more modest. This preliminary study has prompted a full-blown trial to be conducted at Royal Marsden Hospital, in Sutton, England, and the trial began recruiting patients June 4, 2005.[3]

Unlike most treatments discussed in this book, hyperbaric oxygenation may never become widely available, particularly as a home treatment. It involves a huge and very expensive contraption that is unlikely to fit into your guest bedroom, let alone in a bottle or a box.

Nutritional Supplements

The market for supplements is huge. Manufacturers, practitioners, and merchants tout the effectiveness of a wide range of ingredients promising to help in the treatment of lymphedema. But only a few of these have been put through any sort of scientific scrutiny, and you should be able to find them in your local health-food store. And remember that although herbal supplements are usually made with botanical ingredients, they are still drugs; check with your doctor before taking any supplement to make sure it will not interfere with other medications you are currently taking. Here we discuss a few of the supplements promoted as treatments for lymphedema.

Flavonoids

Flavonoids, which occur naturally in many foods, are also known as vitamin P. Foods that are rich in flavonoids include blueberries, onions, apples, grapes, cherries, grapefruit, lemons, oranges, prunes, rose hips, green tea, and the pith of citrus fruits. You can buy flavonoids in health-food stores, but usually they are mixed with other nutrients and sold as bioflavonoids.

Dr. Judith Casley-Smith, founder of the Lymphoedema Association of Australia, says flavonoids can be effective in reducing the swelling of lymphedema, but they work slowly—it may take months to be able to measure a reduction in swelling. Flavonoids are made up of large molecules that are quite bulky for the body to absorb. Because only a small part of the molecule is effective for lymphedema, dosages must be high to be effective (3,000 to 6,000 mg/day).[4] Another complication is the fact that the bioflavonoid complexes normally found in stores yield only about 50 percent flavonoids.

Flavonoids can upset the stomach, so if you decide to try them, start with smaller dosages and let your body adjust before you work up to a level that will reduce the swelling.

Pycnogenols

Pycnogenols (the trade name for a certain class of bioflavonoids) have been used for many years in Europe to reduce swelling in legs and ankles. They hold some promise in treating lymphedema. Pycnogenols come from grape-seed extract and from the French maritime pine (although the company that manufactures them insists that the only real source is the bark of the French maritime pine).[5] You can find both kinds in health-food stores; the ones made from grape-seed extract are usually somewhat less expensive. A trial, sponsored by the National Center for Complementary and Alternative Medicine (NCCAM), is being set up through the University of Wisconsin Comprehensive Cancer Center and the School of Pharmacy to determine the efficacy of Pycnogenols derived from the French maritime pine. As of fall 2004, the study was not yet recruiting patients.[6]

Pycnogenols have no known toxic side effects. They work synergistically with vitamin C to reinforce the vitamin's function in capillary membranes and to strengthen collagen in the capillaries.[5] Recommended dosages differ depending on body weight and on how long the person has been taking them.[7]

Selenium

The mineral selenium is a powerful free-radical scavenger that is believed to increase the benefit of physical therapy for patients who have lymphedema caused by radiation treatment. Good sources for selenium include Brazil nuts, eggs, lean meats, seafood, legumes, and whole grains.[8] Selenium is seldom a cause of toxicity in the body.[9] Again, as with any supplement, before taking selenium discuss its use with your physician.

Benzopyrones (Coumarin)

The most common compounds used to treat lymphedema belong to the chemical family known as the benzopyrones. The smallest of these and the base molecule is called *coumarin*. Practitioners in Australia, India, England, and elsewhere have for some years used benzopyrones with success in treating lymphedema.[10] But in the United States the jury is still out on their effectiveness. A 1999 study published in the *New England Journal of Medicine* found that coumarin had no effect in a group of 140 women with chronic lymphedema.[11] Benzopyrones continue to undergo trials here, and the FDA has not yet approved them.

Coumarin is thought to work by building the body's supply of macrophages, which break down and consume waste cells and high-protein excess fluids. This causes a reduction in the number of protein molecules, waste cells, viruses, and bacteria in the areas of swelling, increasing the possibility for the body to develop alternative lymphatic pathways to remove the waste materials. Dr. Casley-Smith reports that her research shows that coumarin is slow-acting, taking weeks or months to work. It may be administered in any of three ways: orally or in powder or cream form. As a word of caution, the oral application has been deregistered in Australia because a small percentage of patients experienced a type of hepatitis while taking it. The problem seemed to resolve when the benzopyrones were discontinued. No side effects have been reported with the topical use of coumarin, except an occasional mild skin allergy, which goes away if applications are discontinued.[10]

Horsechestnut Herb

Horsechestnut has been shown to be effective in treating venous insufficiency[12] and has been used in Europe for many years to treat both lymphedema of the leg and varicose veins. The University of Wisconsin is endeavoring to scientifically determine its effectiveness in treating lymphedema. A small, preliminary study proved somewhat disappointing; after three months it found no statistical differences among people given the extract and those who took a placebo. However, the researchers were unconvinced of the herb's ineffectiveness and are planning to conduct further investigations. In the fall of 2004 the school was recruiting participants for a larger study.[13]

We're lucky to live in a time when so many medical treatments are available to choose from. It is up to each of us to figure out, and to go for, whatever we believe will make us healthy. The confusion, as well as the beauty, is that there's no absolute way that will work for us all. It's up to us to read, weigh, ask, share and to come up with our own strategy as to what we believe will work for each of us.

24

CONCLUSION

We hope this book helps to answer all of your questions about lymphedema. We hope it assists you in your dealings with doctors and lymphedema therapists. We hope it gives you a sense of control over your future, and a sense that there is a community of people—millions, in fact—who know intimately what you are going through.

Note from Gwen

Writing the first edition of this book was a tremendous experience for me. It helped me to grow as a therapist, required me to learn everything I could about lymphedema, and challenged me in my work with patients. Writing the second edition six years later has been an even greater—and more challenging—learning experience. When I wrote the first edition I had been working with lymphedema for only a short period of time, and I realize now that I did not know very much back then. Still, I wrote *everything* I knew about the condition. Since then I have learned much more and am much more experienced as a therapist. I have worked with hundreds of patients in the last six years.

Much has happened in the lymphedema world since the first edition of this book came out. More research has been conducted, new treatment options and products are available, more schools and organizations have sprung into existence, and more foundations dedicate financial support to lymphedema research. Six years ago, very few articles or books had been published about the condition;

this year, when I typed the word *lymphedema* into the medical-publication search engines, the search yielded almost five hundred articles on the topic. (That number increased to over a thousand when I expanded the search criteria to include radiation-induced scarring and other treatment modalities.) In 1999 only a couple of training options existed in North America for lymphedema therapists; now there are eight or nine such programs. The result is a great increase in the number of trained lymphedema therapists. The number of products and suppliers has also multiplied significantly. The first edition had a Resources section that was only three pages long; the Resources section in this volume is many pages longer than that. It is an exciting time in the sphere of lymphedema treatment.

I continue to feel blessed every day to be able to work with people who have lymphedema. It is an enriching experience for me. Although I do not myself have lymphedema I feel much empathy with those who do. I have a strong desire to help them, teach them, and empower them to take care of themselves. It is my hope that this book will provide lymphedema patients with tools they can put to use immediately, and that doing so will start them on the path of healing.

Note from Jeannie

Like many of the people who shared their personal stories with us, I still have lymphedema. But yearly it fades, in terms of how much thought and effort I devote to it. I continue to be active. I get exercise by walking what feels like half the distance to Singapore every year, I move furniture now and then, and I put in a garden. I eat a good diet and generally live a full and rewarding life. I still bandage when I'm taking on a big project (like cleaning under the couch) and when I fly. And I wear compression garments some days; I even stuff padding under them in particularly stubborn places. I'll admit that last summer I was lazy and my arm got a bit bigger. Gwen's been working on it with me, and the swelling seems to be subsiding. I've also begun to learn that my weight has a lot to do with the state of my arm. When I gain weight my arm responds by swelling even more, and when I lose weight happily the swelling reduces.

I think I'll always be aware of my lymphedema, but no longer as focused on it (read that "obsessed with it") as I once was. It no longer screams for my attention, only hums now and then when I don't pace my life. As I said in the Preface, for now I'm content with that outcome. Knowing what to do about lymphedema has been the key for me, because the knowledge gives me a choice. Every day I make choices in every part of my life, even with lymphedema. And every day my worry about it recedes farther into the distance. My hope is the same for each one of you who reads this book.

Those of us who have lymphedema will likely deal with it for the rest of our lives. What each of us decides to do about it is up to us. We don't choose to have lymphedema, but we don't choose to have cavities in our teeth either, so we floss and we see the dentist regularly. We eat our daily servings of fruits and vegetables. In short, we make efforts in many areas to maintain ourselves and create the best health we can. And so it is with lymphedema. It is a condition that simply requires our care. The better we attend to it, the more we can resume and enjoy the things we love. Isn't that the way it is with all aspects of life?

endnotes

Chapter 1

1. M. Grabois, "Breast Cancer: Post-Mastectomy Lymphedema," *State of the Art Review, Physical Medicine and Rehabilitation Review* 8: 267–277 (1994).

2. Saskia R. J. Thiadens, *Lymphedema: An Information Booklet*, 4th ed. (San Francisco, CA: National Lymphedema Network, 1996).

3. Peter Mortimer, M.D., "The Pathophysiology of Lymphedema," *Cancer Supplement* 83(12): 2798–2802 (15 December 1998).

4. Judith R. Casley-Smith, M.D., *Information about Lymphoedema for Patients*, 6th ed. (Malvern, Australia: Lymphoedema Association of Australia, 1997).

5. A. Bollinger et al., "Aplasia of Superficial Lymphatic Capillaries in Hereditary and Connatal Lymphedema (Milroy's Disease)," *Lymphology* 16:27–30 (1983).

6. National Cancer Institute, Paper on Breast Cancer Treatment, NCI publication, U.S. National Institutes of Health (May 2004).

7. B. Fisher et al., "Five-Year Results of a Randomized Clinical Trial Comparing Total Mastectomy and Segmental Mastectomy with or without Radiation in the Treatment of Breast Cancer," *New England Journal of Medicine* 312(11): 665–673 (1985).

8. J. Armer et al., "Lymphedema Following Breast Cancer Treatment, Including Sentinel Lymph Node Biopsy," *Lymphology* 37(2): 73–91 (2004).

9. Peter Pressman, M.D., "Surgical Treatment and Lymphedema," *Cancer Supplement* 83(12): 2782–2787 (15 December 1998).

10. D. S. Lind, M.D., B. L. Smith, M.D., and W. W. Souba, M.D., "Breast Procedures," in *ACS Surgery: Principles and Practice 2004*, ed. American College of Surgeons (Danbury, CT: WebMD Professional Publishing Inc., 2004) 187–200.

11. U. Veronesi et al., "A Randomized Comparison of Sentinel Node Biopsy with Routine Axillary Dissection in Breast Cancer," *The New England Journal of Medicine* 349: 546–553 (August 2003).

12. W. E. Burak et al., "Sentinel Lymph Node Biopsy Results in Less

Postoperative Morbidity Compared with Axillary Lymph Node Dissection for Breast Cancer," *American Journal of Surgery* 183(1): 23–27 (January 2002).

13. M. Golshan, W. J. Martin, and K. Dowlatshahi, "Sentinel Lymph Node Biopsy Lowers the Rate of Lymphedema when Compared with Standard Axillary Lymph Node Dissection," *The American Surgeon* 69(3): 209–211 (March 2003).

14. C. Ozaslan and B. Kuru, "Lymphedema after Treatment of Breast Cancer," *American Journal of Surgery* 187(1): 69–72 (January 2004).

15. R. H. Ronka et al., "Breast Lymphedema after Breast Conserving Treatment," *Acta Oncologica* 43(6): 551–557 (2004).

16. R. H. Baron et al., "Eighteen Sensations after Breast Cancer Surgery: A Comparison of Sentinel Lymph Node Biopsy and Axillary Lymph Node Dissection," *Oncology Nursing Forum* 29(4): 651–659 (May 2002).

17. K. K. Swenson et al., "Comparison of Side Effects Between Sentinel Lymph Node and Axillary Lymph Node Dissection for Breast Cancer," *Annals of Surgical Oncology* 9(8): 745–753 (October 2002).

18. A. H. Moskovitz et al., "Axillary Web Syndrome after Axillary Dissection," *American Journal of Surgery* 181(5): 434–439 (2001).

19. S. B. Edge et al., "Emergence of Sentinel Node Biopsy in Breast Cancer as Standard of Care in Academic Comprehensive Cancer Centers," abstract, *Breast Diseases: A Yearbook Quarterly* vol. 15, no. 3 (October–December 2004).

20. H. I. Vargas et al., "Lymphatic Tumor Burden Negatively Impacts the Ability to Detect the Sentinel Lymph Node in Breast Cancer," abstract, *Breast Diseases: A Yearbook Quarterly* vol. 15, no. 2 (July–September 2004).

21. Allen G. Meek, M.D., "Breast Radiotherapy and Lymphedema," *Cancer Supplement* 83(12): 2788–2797 (15 December 1998).

22. "Advances in Early-Stage Breast Cancer Treatment," *Harvard Women's Health Watch* vol. 12, no. 2 (October 2004).

23. W. L. Murillo, "Contralateral Breast Management in Breast Reconstruction," *Seminars in Plastic Surgery* 16(1): 77–92 (2002).

24. N. E. Rogers and R. J. Allen, "Radiation Effects on Breast Reconstruction: A Review," *Seminars in Plastic Surgery* 16(1): 19–25 (2002).

25. S. J. Kronowitz et al., "Delayed-immediate Breast Reconstruction," *Plastic Reconstructive Surgery* 113(6): 1617–28 (May 2004).

26. M. Overgaard et al., "Postoperative Radiotherapy in High-Risk Pre-menopausal Women with Breast Cancer Who Receive Adjuvant Chemotherapy," *New England Journal of Medicine* 337:949–955 (1997).

27. J. Ragaz et al., "Adjuvant Radiotherapy and Chemotherapy in Node-Positive Premenopausal Women with Breast Cancer," *New England Journal of Medicine* 337:956–962 (1997).

28. Hester Hill Schnipper, *After Breast Cancer* (New York: Bantam Books, 2003), 52–55.

29. H. Brorson, "Liposuction in Arm Lymphedema Treatment," *Scandinavian Journal of Surgery* 92(4): 287–295 (2003).

30. V. S. Erickson et al., "Arm Edema in Breast Cancer Patients," *Journal of the National Cancer Institute* 93(2): 96–111 (17 January 2001).

31. C. S. Hinrichs et al., "Lymphedema Secondary to Postmastectomy Radiation: Incidence and Risk Factors," *Annals of Surgical Oncology* 11(6): 573–580 (June 2004).

32. S. V. Deo et al., "Prevalence and Risk Factors for Development of Lymphedema Following Breast Cancer Treatment," *Indian Journal of Cancer* 41(1): 8–12 (January–March 2004).

33. M. Golshan, W. J. Martin, and K. Dowlatshahi, "Sentinel Lymph Node Biopsy Lowers the Rate of Lymphedema when Compared with Standard Axillary Lymph Node Dissection," *The American Surgeon* 69(3): 209–211; discussion 212 (March 2003).

34. R. H. Ronka et al., "Breast Lymphedema after Breast Conserving Treatment," *Acta Oncologica* 43(6): 551–557 (2004).

35. Lecture by Nicole Gergich, "Breast and Truncal Edema Management," Reno, NV, 2004 NLN Conference.

36. C. S. Hinrichs et al., "Lymphedema Secondary to Postmastectomy Radiation: Incidence and Risk Factors," *Annals of Surgical Oncology* 11(6): 573–580 (June 2004).

37. M. Deutsch and J. C. Flickinger, "Arm Edema after Lumpectomy and Breast Irradiation," *American Journal of Clinical Oncology* 26(3): 229–231 (June 2003)

38. K. Johansson et al., "Factors Associated with the Development of Arm Lymphedema Following Breast Cancer Treatment: A Match Pair Case-Control Study," *Lymphology* 35(2): 59–71 (June 2002).

39. A. Meek et al., "The Influence of Body Mass Index (BMI) on the Development of Lymphedema in Women Diagnosed with Breast Cancer," *NLN Newsletter* vol. 13, no. 1 (January–March 2001).

Chapter 2

1. Michael Foeldi, M.D., "Treatment of Lymphedema," *Lymphology* 27:1–5 (1994).
2. Judith R. Casley-Smith, M.D., "Signs to Be Aware of for the Onset of Lymphoedema," *Lymphoedema Association of Australia Newsletter* 6 (1996).
3. *Lymphedema* (Bethesda, MD: National Cancer Institute, 1997), 4. Redistributed by University of Bonn Medical Center, 1997.
4. Michael J. Brennan, M.D., "Lymphedema Following the Surgical Treatment of Breast Cancer: A Review of Pathophysiology and Treatment," *Journal of Pain and Symptom Management* 7(2): 112 (1992).
5. Jeanne A. Petrek, M.D., and Melissa Heelan, "Incidence of Breast Carcinoma–Related Lymphedema," *Cancer Supplement* 83(12): 2776–2781 (15 December 1998).
6. Consensus Document of the International Society of Lymphology Executive Committee, "The Diagnosis and Treatment of Peripheral Lymphedema," *Lymphology* 28:113–117 (1995).
7. Michael Foeldi, M.D., "Treatment of Lymphedema," *Lymphology* 27:1–5 (1994).

Chapter 3

1. John W. Hole, Jr., "Lymphatic System," in *Human Anatomy & Physiology*, 6th ed. (Dubuque, IA: William C. Brown Publishers, 1993), 716–723.
2. Walter D. Glanze, Kenneth Anderson, and Lois E. Anderson, eds., "Lymphocyte," in *Signet/Mosby Medical Encyclopedia* (Bergenfield, NJ: Signet New American Library, 1987), 365.
3. Ingrid Kurz, M.D., *Textbook of Dr. Vodder's Manual Lymph Drainage, Volume 2: Therapy*, 2nd ed. (Heidelberg, Germany: Karl F. Haug Publishers, 1989), 43–45.

Chapter 5

1. Kathy LaTour, *The Breast Cancer Companion* (New York: Avon Books, 1993), 380–388.
2. Saskia R. J. Thiadens, and Mitchelle Tanner, "Lymphedema, Breast Cancer and the Brassiere," *National Lymphedema Network Newsletter* vol. 9, no. 3:9 (July 1997).
3. DeCourcy Squire, "Cool Tips for a Hot Summer," *National Lymphedema Network Newsletter* vol. 13, no. 3 (July–September 2001).

4. Peter Mortimer, "Managing Lymphedema," *Clinical and Experimental Dermatology* 20:98–106 (1995).

5. E. Foeldi, M. Foeldi, and L. Clodius, "The Lymphedema Chaos: A Lancet," *Annals of Plastic Surgery* 22(6): 509 (1989).

6. Consensus Document of the International Society of Lymphology Executive Committee, "The Diagnosis and Treatment of Peripheral Lymphedema," *Lymphology* 28:113–117 (1995).

7. Judith R. Casley-Smith, M.D., *Information about Lymphoedema for Patients*, 6th ed. (Malvern, Australia: Lymphoedema Association of Australia, 1997).

8. Judith R. Casley-Smith, M.D., "Tips for Travel," *National Lymphedema Network Newsletter* vol. 12, no. 2 (April–June 2000).

9. Judith Casley-Smith, M.D., and John R. Casley-Smith, M.D., *Information about Lymphoedema for Patients*, 6th ed. (Malvern, Australia: Lymphoedema Association of Australia, 1997), 24.

10. A. H. Mokdad et al., "The Spread of the Obesity Epidemic in the United States," *Journal of the American Medical Association* 282(16): 1519–1522 (October 1999).

11. American Institute of Cancer Research booklet, *A Healthy Weight for Life* E35–WL/F47, http://www.aicr.org/publications/brochures (accessed 8 July 2005).

12. Sonja L. Connor and William E. Connor, M.D., Chapter 1 in *The New American Diet* (New York: Simon and Schuster, 1989).

13. J. A. Petrek et al., "Lymphedema in a Cohort of Breast Carcinoma Survivors 20 Years after Diagnosis," *Cancer* 92:1368–1377 (September 2001).

14. Allen G. Meek, M.D., "Breast Radiotherapy and Lymphedema," *Cancer Supplement* 83(12): 2788–2795 (15 December 1998).

15. M. Deutsch and J. C. Flickinger, "Arm Edema after Lumpectomy and Breast Irradiation," *American Journal of Clinical Oncology* 26(3): 229–231 (June 2003).

16. C. Ozaslan and B. Kuru, "Lymphedema after Treatment of Breast Cancer," *American Journal of Surgery* 187(1): 69–72 (January 2004).

17. J. A. Petrek, News from MSKCC, *Cancer News*, http://www.mskcc.org (June 1998).

18. U.S. Dept. of Health and Human Services, *Diet, Nutrition and Cancer Prevention: A Guide to Food Choices*, NIH publication no. 87-2878 (Washington, DC: Government Printing Office, 1986).

19. American Institute for Cancer Research booklet, *Diet and Health Recommendations for Cancer Prevention* E36–DH/F31.

20. Lecture by Wendy Kohatsu, M.D., "Nutrition and Diet Sense," Women's Health Conference, OHSU Integrative Medicine Clinic, Portland, OR, May 2004.

21. Sonja L. Connor and William E. Connor, M.D., *The New American Diet Cookbook* (New York: Simon and Schuster, 1997).

22. Miles Hassell, M.D., *Optimal Nutrition and Exercise to Reduce the Risk of Breast Cancer,* Providence Health System, 2003.

23. Saskia R. J. Thiadens, "Prevention and Treatment of Lymphedema," *Innovations in Oncology Nursing* 10(3): 62–63 (1994).

24. The Cleveland Clinic Foundation Heart Center, Section of Preventive Cardiology and Rehabilitation, "The Heart-Health Benefits of Chocolate Unveiled," 2004, http://www.clevelandclinic.org/heartcen ter/pub/guide/prevention/nutrition/chocolate.htm (accessed 12 July 2005).

25. A. S. Malin et al., "Intake of Fruits, Vegetables and Selected Micronutrients in Relation to the Risk of Breast Cancer," *Breast Diseases: A Yearbook Quarterly* vol. 15, no. 2 (2004).

26. Michael J. Brennan, M.D., and Linda Miller, "Overview of Treatment Options in Management of Lymphedema," *Cancer Supplement* 83(12): 2821–2827 (15 December 1998).

27. Linda Miller, "Lymphedema: Unlocking the Doors to Successful Treatment," *Innovations in Oncology Nursing* 10(3): 53–62 (1994).

28. Judith R. Casley-Smith, M.D., "Scuba Diving," *Lymphoedema Association of Australia Newsletter* 9 (1995).

Chapter 6

1. H. Wittlinger and G. Wittlinger, *Introduction to Dr. Vodder's Manual Lymph Drainage* (Heidelberg, Germany: Karl F. Haug Publishers, 1986).

2. M. Foeldi, M.D., Ethel Foeldi, M.D., and H. Weissleder, M.D., "Conservative Treatment of Lymphoedema of the Limbs," *Angiology, Journal of Vascular Diseases* 36(3): 171–180 (March 1985).

3. E. Foeldi, M. Foeldi, and L. Clodius, "The Lymphedema Chaos: A Lancet," *Annals of Plastic Surgery* 22(6): 505–515 (1989).

4. Deborah Kelly, *A Primer on Lymphedema*, (Upper Saddle River, NJ: Prentice Hall, 2002), 66.

5. Robert Lerner, M.D., "What's New in Lymphedema Therapy in America?" *International Journal of Angiology* 7(3): 191–196 (1998).

6. Consensus Document of the International Society of Lymphology Executive Committee, "The Diagnosis and Treatment of Peripheral Lymphedema," *Lymphology* 28:113–117 (1995).

7. M. Boris, S.Weindorf, and B. Lasinski, "Persistence of Lymphedema Reduction after Noninvasive Complex Lymphedema Therapy," *Oncology* 11(1): 99–109; discussion 110, 113–114 (January 1997).
8. A. L. Cheville et al., "Lymphedema Management," *Seminars in Radiation Oncology* 13(3): 290–301 (July 2003).
9. Stanley G. Rockson et al., "Diagnosis and Management of Lymphedema," *Cancer Supplement* 83(12): 2882–2885 (1998).
10. Judith R. Casley-Smith, M.D., and John R. Casley-Smith, M.D., "Modern Treatment of Lymphoedema 1. Complex Physical Therapy: The First 200 Australian Limbs," *Australian Journal of Dermatology* 33:61–68 (1992).

Chapter 7

1. A. D. Domar, *Healing Mind, Healthy Woman* (New York: Dell Publishing, 1996).
2. Joan Borysenko, *Minding the Body, Mending the Mind* (New York: Bantam Books, 1988), 62–67.
3. *Managing Stress and Anxiety Workbook* (Kaiser Permanente, 1996).

Chapter 8

1. H. Wittlinger and G. Wittlinger, M.D., *Textbook of Dr. Vodder's Manual Lymph Drainage*, vol. 1, 5th ed., ed. Robert Harris (Brussels, Belgium: Haug International, 1995).
2. Michael Foeldi, M.D., "Treatment of Lymphedema," *Lymphology* 27:1–5 (1994).
3. Joachim E. Zuther, "Understanding Lymphedema," *PT/OT Today* 5(39): 15–22 (1997).
4. Renato Kasseroller, M.D., class notes from Therapy II and III (Victoria, Canada: Dr. Vodder School of North America, August 1997).
5. H. Wittlinger and G. Wittlinger, M.D., *Textbook of Dr. Vodder's Manual Lymph Drainage*, 74.
6. Technique adapted from Nicole Gergich's lecture, "Breast and Truncal Lymphedema," National Lymphedema Network Conference, Reno, Nevada (October 2004).

Chapter 10

1. M. Leidenius et al., "Motion Restriction and Axillary Web Syndrome after Sentinel Node Biopsy and Axillary Clearance in Breast Cancer," *American Journal of Surgery* 185(2): 127–130 (February 2003).

2. A. H. Moskovitz et al., "Axillary Web Syndrome after Axillary Dissection," *American Journal of Surgery* 181(5): 434–439 (2001).

3. Lecture by Jane Kepics, "Physical Therapy Treatment of Axillary Web Syndrome after Breast Cancer Treatment," National Lymphedema Network National Conference, Reno, Nevada (October 2004).

4. Course material, Theresa Schmidt, "Myofascial Release," sponsored by Cross Country University, Portland, Oregon (2004).

5. S. Delanian et al., "Randomized Placebo-Controlled Trial of Combined Pentoxifylline and Tocopherol for Regression of Superficial Radiation-Induced Fibrosis," *Journal of Clinical Oncology* 21(13): 2545–2550 (July 2003).

6. P. Okunieff et al., "Pentoxifylline in the Treatment of Radiation-Induced Fibrosis," *Journal of Clinical Oncology* 22(11): 2207–2213 (June 2004).

Chapter 12

1. H. Wittlinger and G. Wittlinger, M.D., *Textbook of Dr. Vodder's Manual Lymph Drainage*, vol. 1, 5th ed., ed. Robert Harris (Brussels, Belgium: Haug International, 1995), 56.

2. Judith R. Casley-Smith, M.D., "Treatment for Lymphoedema of the Arm: The Casley-Smith Method," *Cancer Supplement* 83(12): 2843–2860 (15 December 1998).

3. Judith Casley-Smith, M.D., and John R. Casley-Smith, M.D., *Information about Lymphoedema for Patients*, 6th ed. (Malvern, Australia: Lymphoedema Association of Australia, 1997), 24.

4. Esther Muscari-Lin, "Truncal Lymphedema," *National Lymphedema Network Newsletter* vol. 16, no. 1 (January–March 2004).

5. Judith Casley-Smith, M.D., and John R. Casley-Smith, M.D., "Compression Bandages in the Treatment of Lymphoedema."

6. Ethel Foeldi, M.D., "Treatment of Lymphedema," *Cancer Supplement* 83(12): 2833–2834 (15 December 1998).

7. Robert Lerner, M.D., "Effects of Compression Bandaging" *Lymphology* 33(2): 169–170 (June, 2000).

8. Linda Miller, "An Introduction to the Management of Breast Cancer Lymphedema: An Integrated Approach," from class notes, Anaheim, California, November 1996.

9. Judith R. Casley-Smith, M.D., and John R. Casley-Smith, M.D., "Modern Treatment of Lymphoedema 1. Complex Physiotherapy: The First 200 Australian Limbs," *Australian Journal of Dermatology* 33:63–69 (1992).

10. Linda Miller, "Lymphedema: Unlocking the Doors to Successful Treatment," *Innovations in Oncology Nursing* 10(3): 53–62 (1994).

11. Susan Harris and Antoinette Megens, "Physical Therapist Management of Lymphedema Following Treatment for Breast Cancer: A Central Review of Its Effectiveness," *Physical Therapy* 78(12): 1302–1311 (1998).

12. Judith R. Casley-Smith, M.D., et al, "Complex Physical Therapy for the Lymphoedematous Arm," *Journal of Hand Surgery* 17(4): 437–441 (August 1992).

13. Claud Regnard, Caroline Badger, and Peter Mortimer, *Lymphoedema: Advice on Treatment*, 2nd ed. (Beaconsfield, England: Beaconsfield Publishers, 1991), 4–8.

Chapter 13

1. Kenzo Kase, Jim Wallis, and Tsuyoshi Kase, *Clinical Therapeutic Applications of the Kinesio Taping Method* (Tokyo, Japan: Kinesio Taping Association, 2003).

2. Kenzo Kase, *Illustrated Kinesio Taping*, 3rd ed., (Albuquerque, NM: Universal Printing and Publishing, 2000).

3. Michael Foeldi, M.D., "Treatment of Lymphedema," *Lymphology* 27:1–5 (1994).

4. E. Foeldi, M. Foeldi, and L. Clodius, "The Lymphedema Chaos: A Lancet," *Annals of Plastic Surgery* 22(6): 509 (1989).

5. A. Szuba, R. Achula, S. Rockson, "Decongestive Lymphatic Therapy for Patients with Breast Carcinoma–Associated Lymphedema. A randomized, prospective study of a role for adjunctive intermittent pneumatic compression," *Cancer* 95(11): 2260–2267 (December 2002).

6. Judith R. Casley-Smith, M.D., and John R. Casley-Smith, M.D., *Information Booklet of the Lymphoedema Association of Australia* (Adelaide, Australia: University of Adelaide, March 1997).

7. Consensus Document of the International Society of Lymphology Executive Committee, "The Diagnosis and Treatment of Peripheral Lymphedema," *Lymphology* 28:113–117 (1995).

8. Guenter Klose, "Treatment Choices for Chronic Extremity Lymphedema," *Physical Therapy Forum* 5(39): 19–22 (19 November 1991).

9. Deborah Kelly, *A Primer on Lymphedema* (Upper Saddle River, NJ: Prentice Hall, 2002).

Chapter 16

1. A. L. Schwartz et al., "Exercise Reduces Daily Fatigue in Women with Breast Cancer Receiving Chemotherapy," *Medical Science, Sports, and Exercise* 33(5): 718–723 (May 2001).

2. J. D. Potter et al., booklet, *Diet and Health Recommendations for Cancer Prevention*, World Cancer Research Fund/American Institute for Cancer Research Expert Panel (2004).

3. David C. Nieman, *The Exercise-Health Connection* (Champaign, IL: Human Kinetics, 1998), 65–67.

4. M. Deutsch and J. C. Flickinger, "Arm Edema after Lumpectomy and Breast Irradiation," *American Journal of Clinical Oncology* 26(3): 229–31 (June 2003).

5. K. Johansson et al., "Factors Associated with the Development of Arm Lymphedema Following Breast Cancer Treatment: A Match Pair Case-Control Study," *Lymphology* 35(2): 59–71 (June 2002).

6. Allen G. Meek, M.D., "Breast Radiotherapy and Lymphedema," *Cancer Supplement* 83(12): 2788 (15 December 1998).

7. Stanley Rockson, M.D., et al., "Diagnosis and Management of Lymphedema," *Cancer Supplement* 83(12): 2882–2885 (15 December 1998).

8. Michael Alter, *Sport Stretch* (Champaign, IL: Human Kinetics, 1990), 1–25.

9. Linda Miller, "Exercise in Management of Breast Cancer–Related Lymphedema," *Innovations in Breast Cancer Care* 3(4): 101–106 (September 1998).

10. Kenneth Cooper, M.D., *The Aerobic Program for Total Well-Being* (New York: M. Evans, 1982), 112.

11. Linda Miller and Michael Brennan, M.D., "Overviews of Treatment Options and Review of the Current Role and Use of Compression Garments, Intermittent Pumps, and Exercise in the Management of Lymphedema," *Cancer Supplement* 83(12): 2821–2827 (15 December 1998).

12. Charles McGarvey III, "Rehab of the Breast Cancer Patient," in *Physical Therapy for the Cancer Patient* (New York: Churchill Livingston, 1990), 67–84.

13. Judith R. Casley-Smith, M.D., "Treatment for Lymphoedema of the Arm: The Casley-Smith Method," *Cancer Supplement* 83(12): 2843–2860 (15 December 1998).

14. Marisa Perdomo, "Conservative Management of Upper Extremity Lymphedema in Cancer Patients," in *Course Notebook, North American Seminars* (Kirkland, WA: 1998).

15. Bob Anderson and Jean Anderson, *Stretching 20th Anniversary* (Bolinas, CA: Shelter Publications, 2000).

16. D. C. McKenzie and A. L. Kalda, "Effect of Upper Extremity Exercise on Secondary Lymphedema in Breast Cancer Patients: A Pilot Study," *Journal of Clinical Oncology* 21(3): 463–466 (February 2003).

17. Linda Miller, "Exercise in Management of Breast Cancer–Related Lymphedema," *Innovations in Breast Cancer Care* 3(4): 101–106 (September 1998).

18. Bonnie Lasinski, "Exercise, Lymphedema and the Limb at Risk," *National Lymphedema Network Newsletter* vol. 13, no. 2 (2001).

19. John R. Casley-Smith, M.D., and Judith R. Casley-Smith, M.D., "Aircraft Flights and Scuba Diving," *National Lymphedema Network Newsletter* 7(3): 8–9 (1995).

20. "Steps for Health" University of Nebraska Cooperative Extension, Lincoln, NE, http://www.lancaster.unl.edu/food/WALK.htm (accessed 12 July 2005).

21. S. Harris and S. Niesen-Vertommen, "Challenging the Myth of Exercise Induced Lymphedema Following Breast Cancer: A Series of Case Reports," *Journal of Surgical Oncology* 74:94–99 (2000).

Chapter 18

1. J. Rovig, M. Miller, and Saskia R. J. Thiadens, "Suggested Guidelines: Questions to Ask when Contacting a Lymphedema Treatment Center," *National Lymphedema Network* special circular (October 1995).

Chapter 19

1. Beverly R. Mirolo et al., "Psychosocial Benefits of Postmastectomy Lymphedema Therapy," *Cancer Nursing* 18(3): 197–205 (1995).

2. Saskia R. J. Thiadens, "18 Steps to Prevention for Upper Extremities," *National Lymphedema Network* special circular (April 1997).

Chapter 21

1. Norman Cousins, *Anatomy of an Illness, as Perceived by the Patient: Reflections on Healing and Regeneration* (New York: Bantam Books, 1981), 27–48.

2. Norman Cousins, *Anatomy of an Illness*, 48.

3. Lee Berk, et al., "Neuroendocrine and Stress Hormone Changes During Mirthful Laughter," *The American Journal of Medical Science* 298(6): 390–396 (December 1989).

4. Lee Berk, "Modulation of Neuroimmune Parameters During the Eustress of Humor Associated Mirthful Laughter," *Journal of Alternative Therapies in Health and Medicine* 7(2): 62–76 (March 2001).

5. Robert R. Provine, *Laughter: A Scientific Investigation* (New York: Viking Penguin, 2000).

6. Kenneth N. Anderson, *The Signet/Mosby Medical Encyclopedia* (New York: Signet New American Library, 1985), 547.

7. Mark Golin, "Natural Tranquilizers: Stress Relief That Works Round the Clock," *Prevention* 47(12): 65–74 (December 1995).

8. Philip J. Hilts, "Health Maintenance Organizations Turn to Spiritual Healing," *The New York Times* 37, 27 December 1995.

9. Cathy Perlmutter, "Break Free from Fatigue Now and Forever," *Prevention* 48(12): 102 (December 1996).

10. Bernie S. Siegel, *Love, Medicine and Miracles* (New York: Harper and Row, 1986), 147–156.

11. G.D. Jacobs, "The Physiology of Mind-Body Interactions: The Stress Response and the Relaxation Response," *Journal of Alternative Complementary Medicine* 7 suppl. 1: S83–92 (2001).

12. Joan Borysenko, *Minding the Body, Mending the Mind* (New York: Bantam Books, 1987), 36.

13. Bernie S. Siegel, *Love, Medicine and Miracles*, 149.

14. Ibid., 150.

15. Ibid., 156.

Chapter 23

1. T. Ashikaga et al., "Support Care," *Cancer* 10(7): 542–548 (October 2002).

2. C. J. Carati et al., "Treatment of Postmastectomy Lymphedema with Low-Level Laser Therapy: A Double Blind, Placebo-Controlled Trial," *Cancer* 98(6): 1114–1122 (15 September 2003).

3. "Clinical Trial: Hyperbaric Oxygen Therapy Compared With Standard Therapy in Treating Chronic Arm Lymphedema in Women Who Have Undergone Radiation Therapy for Early Breast Cancer," http://www.clinicaltrials.gov/ct/gui/show/NCT00077090 (accessed 14 June 2005).

4. Judith R. Casley-Smith, M.D., "Other Oral Products Which May Be Useful in Place of Coumarin," *Lymphoedema Association of Australia Newsletter* 2 (1996).

5. Arnold Pike, "Pycnogenol: A Gift from the Pines," *Let's Live* (reprint), January 1992.

6. Paul Hutson, *Study ID Numbers: R21 AT001724-01*, University of Wisconsin Comprehensive Cancer Center and School of Pharmacy, October 2004.

7. Linda Edwards, "General, Clinical Use of Maritime Pine Pycnogenol," *Fairborne Pycnogenol Monograph* 1:8 (14 July 1997).

8. J. Anderson and B. Deskins, "Selenium," in *The Nutrition Bible* (New York: William Morrow, 1995).

9. Frank Bruns, Oliver Micke, and Michael Bremer, "Current Status of Selenium and Other Treatments for Secondary Lymphedema," *Journal of Supportive Oncology* 1:121–138 (2003).

10. Judith R. Casley-Smith, M.D., "What Is Lymphedema?" in *Information about Lymphoedema for Patients*, 6th ed. (Malvern, Australia: Lymphoedema Association of Australia, 1997), 3.

11. Charles L. Loprinzi et al., "Lack of Effect of Coumarin in Women with Lymphedema after Treatment for Breast Cancer," *The New England Journal of Medicine* 340(5): 346 (4 February 1999).

12. M. H. Pittler and E. Ernst, "Horse-Chestnut Seed Extract for Chronic Venous Insufficiency: A Criteria-Based Systematic Review," *Archives of Dermatology* 134(11): 1356–1360 (November 1998).

13. For information on the study see http://www.medicine.wisc.edu/mainweb/DOMPages.php?section=medicaloncology&page=lymphedema.

glossary

abdomen. The section of the body between the chest and the pelvis.

acupuncture. Traditional Chinese medicine involving insertion of thin needles into the body at specific locations.

adjuvant. Term used to describe an auxiliary treatment. For cancer, it can be chemotherapy, radiation, or hormone therapy that is used to control, destroy, or reduce cancer cells that may have migrated to other areas of the body.

aerobic. Occurring in the presence of oxygen. Aerobic exercise makes the heart and lungs work harder to meet the muscles' need for oxygen.

angion. A single vessel (such as a lymph vessel) that lies between two adjacent valves.

antibiotics. Drugs or other substances that destroy or inhibit the growth of microorganisms.

antibodies. Protein molecules made by the lymph system that fight bacteria, viruses, or other foreign bodies.

antioxidants. Substances that inhibit reactions promoted by oxygen. It is believed that antioxidants play a role in preventing or slowing the growth of some types of cancer.

arterial. Pertaining to the arteries.

arterial capillaries. The smallest blood vessels in the arterial system. Arterial capillaries lie at the very end of arteries, where they connect with venous capillaries. From there, blood without oxygen flows through the veins back to the heart.

artery. A blood vessel that carries oxygenated blood from the heart to the rest of the body.

atrophy. Reduction in the size of a cell, tissue, organ, or other part of the body due to a failure of nutrition to that part. Generally, the wasting away of bodily tissue or an organ.

axilla. The space under the shoulder between the upper part of the arm and the side of the chest (also called the *armpit*).

axillae. Plural of axilla.

axillary node dissection. Surgical procedure involving the removal of lymph nodes in the armpit.

axillary web syndrome. A complication of axillary node dissection in which a band of tissue, made up of scarred veins and lymphatics, runs from the armpit into the arm. Also called *cording*.

B cell. A type of white blood cell, also called a *lymphocyte*, that plays a role in the body's immune response.

B lymphocyte. See *B cell*.

bandaging. In the treatment of lymphedema, the application of a series of specialized low-stretch wraps (as opposed to Ace bandages, which are high-stretch).

belly. See *abdomen*.

benzopyrones. Compounds that stimulate the immune system by helping to remove stagnant protein from bodily tissues, thereby theoretically aiding in the reduction of lymphedema. Also called *coumarin* or *Lodema*. Not currently approved by the FDA.

bilateral mastectomy. Removal of both breasts.

bioflavonoids. Also called *vitamin P*. Bioflavonoids are necessary in the absorption of vitamin C.

biologic. Relating to life and living things. In medicine, a product used in the prevention or treatment of disease.

breast-conservation surgery. Surgical treatment for breast cancer that removes only the tumor, some tissue around the tumor, and axillary lymph nodes. Also called *lumpectomy* or *segmental mastectomy*.

capillaries. The smallest blood vessels, which link the arteries to the veins.

cardiovascular. Having to do with the heart and blood vessels.

CAT scan. See *CT scan*.

cellulitis. Infection of the skin or subcutaneous tissue. Symptoms are heat, redness, pain, and swelling.

chemotherapy. The treatment of disease using highly toxic drugs given intravenously or orally.

chest cavity. The space inside the chest.

chest wall. The area on the trunk above the abdomen and below the collarbone consisting of the sternum and ribs.

circulatory system. The system of blood, blood vessels, lymphatics, and heart related to the circulation of blood and lymph.

collateral. Accessory or secondary, not direct, such as small access vessels.

collateral lymph vessels. Secondary or small branches of the lymph vessels that connect lymph quadrants.

collecting vessels. Vessels in the lymphatic system into which the lymph capillaries drain.

complication. A secondary disease or condition that develops in the course of a primary disease or condition.

complete physical therapy (CPT). Also called *complex decongestive physiotherapy (CDP),* or *combined physiotherapy;* now usually called *decongestive lymphatic therapy.* Therapy used to treat lymphedema. It includes meticulous skin care, lymphatic massage known as *manual lymph drainage (MLD),* compression using special bandages and garments, and exercise.

compression garment. A tightly knit elastic stocking or sleeve that applies pressure to an area of the body to prevent fluid from flowing back and accumulating in the limb.

compression pump. See *vasopneumatic pump.*

compression therapy. See *bandaging.*

compromised. When used with reference to physical systems, those that are endangered or are not working at optimum capacity.

congenital. Present from birth.

congested. To have excessive accumulation of something (e.g., a fluid).

congestive heart failure. A condition in which there is an abnormal accumulation of fluid around the heart.

connective tissue. Tissue that forms the supporting and connecting structures of the body.

constriction. A tightening; the act of making narrower.

contraction. A shortening or a development of tension, as in muscular contraction.

contraindication. Any condition that renders a treatment improper or undesirable.

contralateral. Pertaining to the opposite side.

cording. A complication of axillary lymph node dissection involving a band of tissue, made up of scarred vessels, that runs from the axilla into the arm. Also called *axillary web syndrome.*

cosmetic. Beautifying; made to preserve beauty; made for the sake of appearance.

coumarin. See *benzopyrones.*

CT scan. Computerized axial tomography. A computerized X ray that produces a highly detailed cross-sectional picture of the body's interior.

decongestive therapy. Therapy that reduces the accumulation of fluid in the tissues.

diaphragm. Muscular partition or membrane separating the chest and abdominal cavities.

diaphragmatic breathing. Breathing in which the diaphragm contracts and moves up and down. Sometimes referred to as *belly breathing* or *abdominal breathing.* This type of breathing is believed to aid in the movement of lymph.

dicloxacillin. An antibiotic especially effective in treating skin infections.

distal. Situated away from the point of attachment or origin; for example, the elbow is distal to the shoulder.

diuretics. Drugs or other substances that promote the formation and release of urine.

edema. The presence of abnormally large amounts of fluid in the tissue spaces of the body.

edematous. Having edema.

electromyography. An investigation that tests the electrical potential of muscle and records nerve and muscle function.

enzymes. Complex proteins that are capable of accelerating or producing specific biochemical reactions at body temperature.

Ethafoam roller. A Styrofoam-like roll two to four feet long and four to six inches in diameter, used in exercise.

exacerbate. To increase the severity of or aggravate.

familial. Occurring in or affecting different members of the same family.

fibrosclerotic. Fibers becoming hardened in tissues.

fibrosis. The spreading of fiberlike connective tissue over normal smooth muscle or other tissue.

fibrotic. Having to do with fibrosis; harder than normal tissue, often referred to as *scar tissue.*

filament. A thin fiber such as that attaching from the connective tissue to the initial lymphatic vessel to open the flaps of the vessel so it will take in lymph

filariasis. Infestation of the lymphatics by a mature larvae of the parasite *Wuchereria bancrofti.*

filter. To strain water or other fluid to separate out particulate matter.

filtration. Outflowing of fluids in the body, as when blood and its components filter into interstitial tissues through arterial capillaries.

flavonoids. Having to do with flavones, crystalline compounds found in many plants. Flavonoids are believed to aid in the processing of proteins, bacteria, and other foreign matter in the body.

genetic. Pertaining to birth or origin, inherited.

gymnastic ball. A large ball used during exercise, particularly to gain and maintain strength and flexibility. Also called *therapy ball.*

hypoallergenic. Not likely to cause an allergic response.

immune system. The body's ability to protect itself from disease, organisms, other foreign bodies, and cancers. The lymphatic system is a part of the immune system.

immunity. The capacity to resist a disease, organism, other foreign body, or cancer.

indication. That which indicates the proper treatment. A circumstance that shows the cause, pathology, or treatment of a disease.

inflammation. A response by the body to cells damaged by injury or irritation. The signs of inflammation are usually redness, pain, heat, and swelling.

initial lymph vessels. The fingerlike projections into the interstitial tissue where the lymph enters the lymphatic system; the beginning of the lymph system. Also called *lymph capillaries.*

in situ. Confined to the site of origin without invading neighboring tissues.

interstitial. The space between the body's tissues.

interventions. Actions intended to prevent an occurrence or maintain or alter a condition.

invasive breast cancer. Breast cancer that has spread into the nonbreast tissue.

involved limb. The arm or leg that has lymphedema.

involved quadrant. The lymphatic-drainage quarter of the body that has lymphedema.

Keflex. The trademark name for an antibiotic that is particularly effective in treating infections of the skin.

Kinesio Tex Tape. The elasticized cloth tape used in the Kinesio Taping Method.

Kinesio Taping Method. The application of a special tape to the skin to stimulate the movement of fluid and soften fibrosis.

kyphotic thoracic spine. Curvature of the thoracic spine from the lower cervical area to the upper lumbar. Characterized by vertebra with ribs attached.

lumpectomy. Surgical removal of a breast tumor, a small area of surrounding tissue, and some axillary lymph nodes. Also called *breast-conservation surgery*.

lymph. A thin, pale, clear, yellowish fluid that bathes the body's tissues, passes into lymphatic channels and ducts, and is filtered by the lymph nodes before it is discharged into the blood by way of the thoracic duct.

lymphangiography. X-ray examination of the lymph glands and vessels after injection of a dye.

lymphangiosarcoma. A rare cancer of the lymphatic system.

lymphangitis. A bacterial infection of the lymphatic system.

lymphatic capillary. Smallest lymph-carrying vessel.

lymphatic massage. A specialized, very gentle massage that stimulates the lymphatic system and moves fluid from an area of the body that is unable to process it to an area that can. Also called *manual lymph drainage*.

lymphatics. Having to do with lymph; also, tissue relating to the lymph glands, lymph vessels, or lymphocytes.

lymphatic system. A vast and complex network of capillaries, thin vessels, valves, ducts, and nodes that is responsible for filtering lymph fluid and carrying it from the tissues to the thoracic duct, which returns the fluid to the blood. Also plays a role in protecting the body against illness.

lymphatic vessels. Vessels that convey lymph.

lymphedema. Swelling caused by an accumulation of lymphatic fluid in the tissues.

lymphedema, congenital. Lymphedema that is present from birth.

lymphedema, praecox. Primary lymphedema that develops during adolescence.

lymphedema, primary. Lymphedema that has no known cause.

lymphedema, secondary. Lymphedema that occurs after compromise to the lymphatic system by surgery, trauma, radiation, or infection.

lymphedema, tarda. Primary lymphedema that develops in adulthood, usually after age thirty-five.

lymph nodes. Small oval structures that remove waste from the body's tissues, filter lymph, fight infection, and produce white blood cells. The human body contains five hundred to fifteen hundred lymph nodes, usually clumped in groups in the neck, axilla, groin, abdomen, and trunk.

lymphocytes. Specialized, small white blood cells that increase in number during infection and customize themselves to destroy foreign proteins and to fight the infection.

lymphology. The study of lymphatics.

lymphoscintigraphy. A diagnostic technique that creates a two-dimensional picture of lymph vessels by using radioisotopes.

lymphostasis. Pooling or stagnation of the lymph fluid.

macrophages. Large, wandering cells that ingest microorganisms or other cells and foreign particles.

malignancy. Cancerous growth.

mammary glands. Milk-producing glands located in the breast.

manual lymph drainage (MLD). A special massage technique that transports lymphatic fluid from an area of the body with congestion or edema to an area with functioning lymphatics. Used to treat lymphedema.

mastectomy. Surgical removal of one breast, some surrounding tissue, and axillary lymph nodes on the same side. Also known as *modified radical mastectomy.*

metabolism. The chemical change in living cells by which energy is provided for vital processes.

metastasis. The spread of cancer cells to distant parts of the body, usually through the lymph system or blood vessels.

microbe. A minute organism or bacteria. A germ.

Milroy's disease. Form of hereditary lymphedema, present at birth, in which there is an absence of initial lymph vessels.

MLD. See *manual lymph drainage.*

moxibustion. Chinese herbal treatment.

MRI. Magnetic resonance imaging. Test using electromagnets, frequency waves, and a computer to provide an image.

myofasical tissue. A sheet of tissue lying just beneath the skin which surrounds the muscular tissue, separating the layers.

myofascial release technique. A technique of applying gentle, sustained pressure to the skin to stretch scar tissue.

muscle hyperactivity. Excessive activation of muscles.

National Lymphedema Network (NLN). The main clearinghouse of information on lymphedema in the United States.

neoadjuvant. Refers to chemotherapy that is given to shrink a tumor before its surgical removal.

nodes. See *lymph nodes.*

oncologist. A doctor specializing in the study and treatment of cancer.

oncology. The study of cancer and its treatment.

oxygenate. To saturate with oxygen.

pain threshold. The point at which pain receptors are stimulated and one feels pain.

palpate. To check the texture, size, and location of parts of the body with the hands.

paraspinal. Adjacent or near to the spinal column.

pectoral. Area of the body on the chest wall going from the shoulder to the underlying breast.

PET scan. Positron emission tomography scan. A diagnostic X-ray test to preoperatively assess axillary node involvement for the staging of breast cancer.

peristalsis. The rhythmic wave of contraction along the digestive tract, the purpose of which is to propel its contents.

pH. The scale indicating the level of acidity or alkalinity.

physical therapy. The treatment of disorders by physical means.

physiologic. The workings of the human body.

physiology. The study of the workings of the human body.

pitting edema. An indentation that will take some time to fill in, caused by pressure to an area of swelling.

predisposition. A latent susceptibility to disease that may be activated under certain conditions.

pressure stroke. The massage stroke that applies pressure to the tissue in a specific direction. Compare *release stroke.*

primary lymphedema. See *lymphedema, primary.*

prophylactic. Guarding from or preventing disease; preventive.

prosthesis. An apparatus that replaces a part of the body.

proteins. A very large and complex group of compounds that are composed of amino acids and are essential to tissue growth and repair.

proximal. Nearest to the trunk of the body.

pycnogenol. A bioflavonoid that is found in the bark of the French maritime pine and in grape seed. It is believed to help circulation and to aid in maintaining healthy arteries.

quadrant. Quarter, section.

radiation fibrosis. Hardening or thickening of tissue caused by radiation.

radiation oncology. The medical field that treats cancer through radiation.

radical mastectomy. Surgical treatment for breast cancer in which the breast tissue, muscles of the chest wall, a portion of skin, and all the lymph nodes under the arm are removed. Also known as the *Halsted radical mastectomy.*

radiotherapy. Treatment of disease by means of X rays or radioactive substances.

reconstructive surgery. Surgery to construct again something that has been removed, e.g., breast reconstructive surgery after mastectomy.

rehabilitation. To restore to the former state of normal form and function after injury or illness.

release stroke. The massage stroke in which no pressure is being applied, but the hand is moving into a position to prepare for the pressure stroke that will follow. Compare *pressure stroke.*

resorption. Uptake, as in uptake of fluid from interstitial tissue into venous capillaries.

sclerosed. Thickened or hardened, such as a body part.

secondary lymphedema. See *lymphedema, secondary.*

segmental compression. Pressure applied sequentially, causing the lymphatic fluid to circulate out of the affected limb.

selenium. A chemical element that resembles sulfur; also an essential dietary mineral.

self-massage. Massage done by oneself, for example to stimulate lymph nodes and to move lymph.

sentinel node. The first lymph node to receive lymphatic drainage from a tumor.

sentinel node biopsy. Surgical procedure in which the breast tumor is injected with dye, which travels along the lymphatic vessels to the first node in the axilla. That node is removed and evaluated for cancer. If the node is negative, axillary node dissection can be avoided.

sequential gradient pump. See *vasopneumatic pump.*

seroma. A pocket of fluid that accumulates around a surgical site.

shoulder girdle. The body's support for and method of maintaining the shoulder. Consisting of shoulder blade, clavicle, and upper arm, and muscles and ligaments related to those.

simple mastectomy. A mastectomy that removes only the breast tissue.

staging. Assessing the degree of development of a disease. A stage is a distinct phase in the course of disease; for example, stage I or stage II breast cancer.

stationary circles. In massage, circular motions done in one spot on the body (such as the base of the neck) with the flat tips of the fingers.

stretch reflex. A reflex contraction of a muscle in response to a passive stretch.

subclavian. Located under the collarbone.

supraclavicular. Situated above the collarbone.

systemic. Pertaining to or affecting the body as a whole.

sweep. In massage, a gentle pushing in the direction in which lymph fluid is to flow.

T cell. A small white blood cell that has various functions in the immune system. Nicknamed "killer cell" because it secretes special compounds that assist B cells in destroying foreign proteins. Also called *T lymphocyte.*

tamoxifen. A drug used in the treatment of certain types of breast cancer that blocks the action of estrogen.

Theraband. A stretchy band used during certain exercises to increase strength and circulation.

therapy ball. A large, air-filled ball used while exercising. Can assist in building flexibility and strength. Also called *gymnastic ball.*

thoracic duct. The main collecting duct of the lymphatic system, receiving lymph from the left side of the head, neck, and chest, the left upper limb, and the entire body beneath the ribs. It is located high in the abdomen and runs up through the thorax (chest).

thorax. The chest area.

thrombosis. The development or presence of a clot or plug in a blood vessel.

thymocyte. A cell of the thymus.

thymus. A gland in the chest, located behind the sternum and between the lungs. It is a central gland of the lymphatic system, housing lymphocytes and macrophages.

T lymphocyte. See *T cell.*

transport capacity. The amount of lymph fluid the lymphatic system is able to carry. Fluid continuously moves from the bloodstream into the tissues and back into the bloodstream. If the transport capacity is exceeded, the lymph fluid will back up, causing lymphedema.

uninvolved limb. The limb that does not have lymphedema.

upper extremity. The arm.

vascular. Pertaining to vessels.

vasopneumatic pump. A pump attached to a sleeve that encases the involved arm or leg and segmentally distributes pressure from distal to proximal in order to move lymph out of the limb. Also called a *sequential gradient pump.*

VEGF-C. Vascular endothelial growth factor C (a hormone). Recent research indicates that VEGF-C may improve function of the lymphatics after cancer.

veins. Vessels that transport blood without oxygen back to the heart.

venous. Having to do with veins.

venous capillaries. Small veins that connect with arterial capillaries.

venous insufficiency. Abnormally low circulation of blood returning from the legs to the trunk. Can cause fluid buildup, pain, varicose veins, and ulceration.

vessel. A small tube in the body that carries fluids such as blood or lymph.

visualization. The achievement of a visual impression of an object; the picturing of something in one's mind.

waste product. Debris that is of no use to the bodily system.

watersheds. The invisible lines dividing the various lymphatic sections of the body. The vertical watershed is marked by the sternum, the horizontal ones by the waistline and the collarbone.

selected bibliography

Also see the Recommended Reading List that follows.

Beers, Mark H., and Robert Berkow, M.D., eds. *The Merck Manual of Diagnosis and Therapy*, Centennial ed. Whitehouse Station, NJ: Merck Research Laboratories, 1999.

Casley-Smith, Judith R., M.D. *Information about Lymphoedema for Patients*, 6th ed. Malvern, Australia: Lymphoedema Association of Australia, 1997.

Casley-Smith, Judith R., M.D. *Modified Treatment for Lymphoedema*, 8th ed. Malvern, Australia: Lymphoedema Association of Australia, 1999.

Domar, Alice, and Henry Dreher. *Healing Mind, Healthy Woman*. New York: Bantam Doubleday Dell Publishing, 1997.

Dorland, W.A. Newman, ed. *Dorland's Illustrated Medical Dictionary*, 24th ed. Philadelphia, PA: W.B. Saunders, 1994.

Foeldi, Michael, and Ethel Foeldi. *Lymphoedema: Methods of Treatment and Control*, 5th ed. New York: Gustav Fischer Verlag, 1991.

Foeldi, Michael, and Roman Strößenreuther. *Foundations of Manual Lymph Drainage*, 3rd ed. St. Louis, MO: Elsevier Mosby, 2005.

Glanze, Walter D., Kenneth N. Anderson, and Lois E. Anderson, eds. *The Signet Mosby Medical Encyclopedia*. New York: Signet/New American Library, 1987.

Hole, John W., Jr. "Lymphatic System." In *Human Anatomy/Physiology*, 6th ed., 716–723. Dubuque, IA: William C. Brown Publishers, 1993.

Halverstadt, Amy, and Andrea Leonard. *Essential Exercises for Breast Cancer Survivors*. Boston, MA: The Harvard Common Press, 2000.

Kase, Kenzo. *Illustrated Kinesio Taping*, 3rd ed. Albuquerque, NM: Universal Printing and Publishing, 2000.

Kase, Kenzo, Tsuyoshi Kase, and Jim Wallis. *Clinical Therapeutic Applications of the Kinesio Taping Method*. Tokyo, Japan: Kinesio Taping Association, 2003.

Kelly, Deborah G. *A Primer on Lymphedema*. Upper Saddle River, NJ: Prentice Hall, 2002.

Lebed-Davis, Sherry. *Thriving after Breast Cancer.* New York: Broadway Books, 2002.

Schnipper, Hester Hill. *After Breast Cancer.* New York: Bantam Dell, 2003.

Thiadens, Saskia R. J. *Lymphedema: An Information Booklet,* 4th ed. San Francisco, CA: National Lymphedema Network, 1996.

Thomas, Clayton L., ed. *Taber's Cyclopedic Medical Dictionary,* 18th ed. Philadelphia, PA: F. A. Davis, 1997.

Zuckweiler, Rebecca. *Living in the Postmastectomy Body.* Point Roberts, WA: Hartley and Marks Publishers, 1998.

Recommended Reading

American Institute of Cancer Research. *A Healthy Weight for Life.* Booklet E35-WL/F47. Washington, DC. Retrieved 7 July 2005 from http:www.aicr.org/publications/brochures/online/wl.htm.

American Institute of Cancer Research. *Diet and Health Recommendations for Cancer Prevention.* Booklet E36-DH/F31. Washington, DC. An order form for this publication can be found at http://www.aicr.org/information/hp/hpb.pdf.

Anderson, Bob, and Jean Anderson. *Stretching,* 20th anniversary ed. Bolinas, CA: Shelter Publications, 2000.

Casley-Smith, Judith R., M.D. *Information about Lymphoedema for Patients,* 6th ed. Malvern, Australia: Lymphoedema Association of Australia, 1997.

Connor, Sonja L., and William E. Connor. *The New American Diet Cookbook.* New York: Simon and Schuster, 1989.

Devi, Nischala Joy. *The Healing Path of Yoga.* New York: Three Rivers Press, 2000.

Domar, Alice, and Henry Dreher. *Healing Mind, Healthy Woman.* New York: Bantam Doubleday Dell Publishing, 1997.

Gallagher-Mundy, Chrissie. *Essential Guide to Stretching.* New York: Random House Value Publishing, 1996.

Halverstadt, Amy, and Andrea Leonard. *Essential Exercises for Breast Cancer Survivors.* Boston, MA: The Harvard Common Press, 2000.

Harmon-Jenkins, Nancy. *The Mediterranean Diet Cookbook.* New York: Bantam Books, 1994.

Hobler, Deborah. *No Less a Woman: Femininity, Sexuality & Breast Cancer,* 2nd ed. Alameda, CA: Hunter House Publishers, 1995.

Hoffman, Lisa, with Alison Freeland. *The Healing Power of Movement.* Cambridge, MA: Perseus Publishing, 2002.

Lasater, Judith. *Living Your Yoga: Finding the Spiritual in Everyday Life.* Berkeley, CA: Rodmell Publishing, 2000.

Lebed-Davis, Sherry. *Focus on Healing Through Movement and Dance for the Breast Cancer Survivor.* Videotape. Morro Bay, CA: Enhancement, Inc., 1998.

Lebed-Davis, Sherry, and Stephanie Gunning. *Thriving after Breast Cancer.* New York: Broadway Books, 2002.

McGinn, Kerry A., and Pamela J. Haylock. *Women's Cancers: How to Prevent Them, How to Treat Them, How to Beat Them,* 3rd ed. Alameda, CA: Hunter House Publishers, 2003.

Mitchell, Rita, Bob Arnot, and Barbara Sutherland. *The Breast Health Cookbook.* New York: Little, Brown and Company, 2001.

O'Brien, Paddy. *A Gentler Stretch, The Yoga Book for Women.* London: Thorsons, 1992.

Ratner, Elaine. *The Feisty Woman's Breast Cancer Book.* Alameda, CA: Hunter House Publishers, 1999.

Ricks, Delthia. *Breast Cancer Basics and Beyond: Treatment, Resources, Self-Help, Good News, Updates.* Alameda, CA: Hunter House Publishers, 2005.

Schnipper, Hester Hill. *After Breast Cancer.* New York: Bantam Dell, 2003.

Stumm, Diana. *Recovering from Breast Surgery: Exercises to Strengthen Your Body and Relieve Pain.* Alameda, CA: Hunter House Publishers, 1995.

Thiadens, Saskia R. J. *Lymphedema: An Information Booklet,* 4th ed. San Francisco, CA: National Lymphedema Network, 1996.

Thiadens, Saskia R. J. *18 Steps for Preventing Lymphedema.* San Francisco, CA: National Lymphedema Network, 1997.

U.S. Dept of Health and Human Services. *Diet, Nutrition and Cancer Prevention: A Guide to Food Choices.* NIH publication no. 87-2878. Washington, DC: Government Printing Office, 1986.

Zuckweiler, Becky. *Living in the Postmastectomy Body.* Point Roberts, WA: Hartley and Marks Publishers, 1998.

resources

Technology, help, and support for lymphedema sufferers have come a long way. Besides the intrepid Saskia Thiadens and the National Lymphedema Network, who have been speaking on patients' behalf for several years, new support groups, certifying agencies, therapists, and products continue to spring into existence. This section lists many of them.

Associations and Organizations

The National Lymphedema Network (NLN)
Latham Square
1611 Telegraph Ave., Suite 111
Oakland CA 94612-2138   Infoline: (800) 541-3259
E-mail: nln@lymphnet.org   Website: www.lymphnet.org
This nonprofit organization was founded in 1988 by Saskia R. J. Thiadens, R.N., to provide education and guidance to lymphedema patients, health-care professionals, and the general public. Services include:
* Referral to lymphedema treatment centers and health-care professionals. The website lists therapists certified to perform treatment for lymphedema. Note that not all therapists register with the NLN; there may be additional qualified therapists in your area.
* Many publications available to the public about lymphedema and its treatment.
* Quarterly newsletters with information about medical and scientific developments, support groups, pen pals, updated resource guides, and more.
* Educational courses for health-care professionals and patients.
* An extensive computer database.
* Biennial international conferences.

Lymphology Association of North America (LANA)
P.O. Box 466
Wilmette IL 60091   (773) 756-8971
E-mail: lana@telusys.net   Website: www.clt-lana.org
Finding qualified lymphedema therapists was once a daunting task. LANA was founded in 2001 in response to the need for minimum competency standards for the treatment of lymphedema. LANA is a nonprofit corporation whose members are health-care professionals experienced in

the field of lymphology and lymphedema, including physicians, nurses, massage therapists, physical therapists, and occupational therapists. To become LANA certified, therapists must pass rigorous standards, including 135 hours of CDT training; one year of documented experience after the training; and 180 hours of college-level human anatomy, physiology, and/or pathology. Therapists must recertify through LANA every six years.

The Lymphoedema Association of Australia (LAA)
94 Cambridge Terrace
Malvern, SA 5061, Australia
+61-8-8271-2198, +61-8-8271-8776, fax
Website: www.lymphoedema.org.au
Email: Casley@intcrnode.on.net
Chair: Judith R. Casley-Smith, Ph.D., M.A., M.D. (h.c), Prof.(h.c. multi). The LAA is a worldwide leader in the research and treatment of lymphedema. Founded in 1982 by Drs. John R. and Judith R. Casley-Smith, its mission is to perform research; to aid patients; and to educate patients, therapists, and doctors. It has also been a leader in research and education on the use and benefits of decongestive lymphatic therapy and on the effects of benzopyrones on lymphedema.

The LAA has available a library of pamphlets, videos, and newsletters. Its most recent publications include *Modern Treatment for Lymphoedema, High-Protein Oedemas and the Benzo-Pyrones* (for doctors and therapists), *Information about Lymphoedema for Patients,* and *Exercises for Patients with Lymphoedema of the Arm and a Guide to Self-Massage and Hydrotherapy.* It also offers music tapes to accompany the exercise routines, as well as videos on exercises, causes of edema, benzopyrones, and microcirculation.

International Society of Lymphology
University of Arizona, College of Medicine, Department of Surgery
P.O. Box 245063
1501 N. Campbell Ave.
Tucson AZ 85724-5063   (520) 626-6118
E-mail: lymph@u.arizona.edu   Website: www.u.arizona.edu/~witte
Secretary General: Marlys H. Witte, M.D.
Founded to advance and disseminate knowledge in the field of lymphology, establish relations between researchers and clinicians, further the exchange of ideas among lymphologists, and strengthen experimental and clinical investigation into lymphedema.

Lymphatic Research Foundation (LRF)
100 Forest Dr.
East Hills NY 11548   (516) 625-9675, (516) 625-9410 fax

E-mail: lrf@lymphaticresearch.org
Website: www.lymphaticresearch.org
Founder and President: Wendy Chaite, Esq.
A not-for-profit organization dedicated to supporting and promoting lymphatic research. Its mission is to foster an interdisciplinary field of research that provides health benefits to all individuals and in particular leads to therapeutic advances and a cure for lymphatic disease, lymphedema, and related disorders. LRF's immediate goal is to increase both public awareness and public and private funding for lymphatic research.

The North American Vodder Association of Lymphatic Therapy (NAVALT)
833 Independence Dr.
Longmont CO 80501   (888) 4NAVALT (888-462-8258)
Website: www.navalt.org
A nonprofit association for therapists who are certified in the Dr. Vodder method of manual lymph drainage and for people who have lymphedema or lymphatic diseases. NAVALT conducts a yearly educational conference open to everyone. It also publishes a newsletter four times per year containing information and case studies about diseases of the lymph system.

Online Support Group
Lymphedema People   www.lymphedemapeople.com
A comprehensive web forum and clearinghouse of information for people concerned about lymphedema.

Lymphedema Training Programs (North America)

Dr. Vodder School of North America
P.O. Box 5701
Victoria BC V8R 6S8, CANADA   (250) 522-9862, (250) 598-9841, fax
Website: www.vodderschool.com
Director: Robert Harris, HND, RMT, CLT-LANA
Offers training programs for therapists throughout Canada and the United States. It can also provide information about MLD-certified therapists in your area. Its mission is to provide the highest-quality education in the Dr. Vodder method of manual lymph drainage and combined decongestive therapy and to ensure the continuing competence of practitioners trained by the Dr. Vodder School.

Academy of Lymphatic Studies
11632 High St., Suite A
Sebastian FL 32958   (772) 589-3355
Website: www.acols.com
Director: Joachim E. Zuther, CI

Medical Director: Michael King, M.D., FACP, FACC
Offers extensive training programs and certification for lymphedema treatment, including training of medical doctors, physical therapists, nurses, occupational therapists, and massage therapists (massage therapists need to fulfil certain criteria for entry). Also maintains a listing of and reference service for therapists who have completed the program.

CLT-Courses
115 Leyden St.
Decatur GA 30030
(800) 642-3629, (404) 377-9883, ext. 2
E-mail: CLTcourses@cs.com
Director: DeCourcy Squire, P.T., CLT, CS-CI
A Casley-Smith affiliate in the U.S. Offers a 135-hour, seventeen-day training program that is open to doctors, nurses, physical and occupational therapists, massage therapists, and physical and occupational therapy assistants.

Lymphedema Therapy Boris-Lasinski School
77 Froehlich Farm Blvd.
Woodbury NY 11797   (516) 364-2200, (516) 364-1844, fax
Founders and Directors: Marvin Boris, M.D., Bonnie B. Lasinski, P.T.
A Casley-Smith affiliate. Physicians and physical therapists at the school have been trained in complex lymphedema therapy (CLT) by Drs. John and Dr. Judith Casley-Smith of Australia. Besides providing training for lymphedema therapists, the school operates a practice dedicated to the diagnosis, treatment, and management of individuals with either primary or secondary lymphedema, including lymphedema complicated by open wounds. Patient education and self-care are emphasized.

Klose Training and Consulting
110 Highway 35
Red Bank NJ 07701   (866) 621-7888, (732) 530-7888
(732) 530-2802, fax
Website: www.klosetraining.com   E-mail: info@klosetraining.com
Director: Lawrence N. Sampson, M.D.
Provides training in manual lymph drainage and complete decongestive therapy with a 135-hour, twelve-day course. Maintains the highest standards of training by drawing upon its staff members' many years of practical experience, monitoring the latest developments in MLD-CDT treatments, and providing students with the best educational materials available.

The Upledger Institute
11211 Prosperity Farms Rd., Suite D-325
Palm Beach Gardens FL 33410   (561) 622-4334

Website: www.upledger.com
Directors: Bruno Chikly, M.D., Renee Romero, R.N.
Offers a 140-hour, eighteen-day training program in lymphedema therapy. Its Health Resource Center focuses on continuing-education programs, clinical research, and therapeutic services using lymph drainage therapy (LDT). The center employs more than seventy on-site professional and clinical staff, plus more than two thousand trained instructors, teaching assistants, and course facilitators in North, Central, and South America, Europe, India, Asia, the Middle East, New Zealand, and Australia. Also makes a wide selection of support and reference materials available to the public.

Norton School of Lymphatic Therapy
326 Broad St.
Red Bank NJ 07701   (866) 445-9674, (732) 842-4414
E-mail: info@nortonschool.com   Website: www.nortonschool.com
Director: Andrea Cheville, M.D.
In the tradition of the Foeldi method of complete decongestive therapy (CDT) this school trains medical doctors, physical therapists and their assistants, occupational therapists and their assistants, registered nurses, and nationally certified massage therapists to become experts in the treatment of pathologies related to the lymphatic system.

Centro de Estudios Linfáticos
9945 NW 47 Terr.
Doral FL 33178-1938
(305) 477-6409, USA+55-2614-5118, Mexico
E-mail: StudyMLD@aol.com
Director: Monika Keller, NCTMB, CLT-LANA
Offers clinical therapy for lymphedema and related diseases, a fully accredited training program in manual lymphatic drainage and complete decongestive therapy, and specialty seminars in the areas of bandaging, pediatrics, and wound care. The clinic is staffed by certified lymphedema therapists, including bilingual therapists. Classes are taught by European instructors trained in the Foeldi method. Training programs are offered at various locations throughout Mexico, both in Spanish and English.

Lymphedema Training Programs (Outside North America)
Dr. Vodder Schule-Walchsee
Alleestrasse 30, A-6344 Walchsee, Tyrol, AUSTRIA
+43-5374-5245-0, +43-5374-5245-4, fax
Website: www.vodderschule.com
The Vodders pioneered the manual lymph drainage (MLD) system. In 1967 the Society for Dr. Vodder's Manual Lymph Drainage was founded with the aim to scientifically substantiate the effects of MLD and create

courses of study for various professional groups. The school now offers basic and advanced training in the original Vodder method at various locations in North America. Classes in Walchsee are usually given in German, but at least one class yearly is taught in English. The Vodder School maintains lists of Vodder-certified therapists throughout the world.

The Foeldi School-Privateschule Foeldi GMBH
Clinic of Lymphology
Rosslehofweg 2-6
79856 Hinterzarten, GERMANY
+49-7652-1240, +49-7652-124116, fax
Website: www.foeldiklinik.de
Directors: Dr. Michael Foeldi, Dr. Ethel Foeldi
The Foeldi Clinic and School was started in the early 1980s. It trains occupational and physical therapists, massage therapists, physicians, and nurses. Recently it has added classes geared to English-speaking therapists and to physicians. The Clinic offers intensive residential treatment programs for people with lymphedema.

The Casley-Smith School
94 Cambridge Terr.
Malvern, AUSTRALIA 5061
+61 8 8271-2198, +61-8-8271-8776, fax
E-mail: Casley@internode.on.net   Website: www.lymphoedema.org.au
Director: Dr. Judith Casley-Smith
Offers a training program in complete decongestive therapy. Courses in Australia were suspended in October 2004 due to unforeseen circumstances. Check the website for current information.

Inpatient Lymphedema Treatment Program

Providence St. Peter Hospital
Inpatient Lymphedema Clinic
Department of Physical Medicine and Rehabilitation
413 Lilly Rd. NE MS01B03
Olympia WA 98506
Questions to Anita Wilkinson, R.N., at (888) 491-9480, ext. 37646.

Suppliers and Distributors of Lymphedema Products

The following list is by no means complete and your lymphedema therapist may also be able to direct you to local suppliers. We do not endorse or recommending any specific company or product; the list is simply an attempt to present a broad spectrum of products that may be useful for the management of your lymphedema.

Bandaging Products

Bandages Plus   (800) 770-1032
A distributor of compression therapy supplies. It provides a complete line of bandages, foams and paddings, Kinesio Tex Tape, skin- and wound-care products, compression garments, and educational materials and classes. Several of its staff are lymphedema therapists.

North American Rehabilitation   (800) 300-5512
Website: www.healthclick.com/nar_main.cfm
Carries a full line of compression therapy supplies for lymphedema treatment. It also offers educational products. The company says its products can arrive anywhere in the continental United States within three business days of ordering.

Bandages Direct   (866) 99-LYMPH (866-995-9674)
Website: www.bandagesdirect.com
Owned by lymphedema therapists and provides a wide selection of bandages, compression garments, and lymphatic health products.

Lymphawrap   (480) 661-1820
E-mail: lymphawraps@qwest.net
Website: www.lymphawrap.com
Distributes a variety of lymphedema products, including Kinesio Tex Tape, several brands of bandages, gloves, foam, and foam wrapping. The company is also the exclusive distributor of the Lymphawrap, a synthetic tubular stockinette known for its softness and coolness.

Academy Bandages   (800) 863-5935
Website: www.acols.com/store.html
A subsidiary of the Academy of Lymphatic Studies; provides a comprehensive line of lymphedema-management products, including brand-name bandages, foams, compression garments, and accessory items. It also offers educational materials.

Lohmann and Rauscher   (800) 279-3863
Offers a complete line of quality bandaging products and accessories, including Rosidal short-stretch bandages and Komprex foam padding.

Kinesio Tex Tape
Website: www.kinesiotaping.com
Kinesio Tex Tape is an elastic, cotton, fabric tape developed in Japan by Kenzo Kase, D.C. The tape stimulates the movement of lymphatic and interstitial fluids by creating a gentle massage that reduces edema and pain and improves the return of normal sensation.

Compression Garments

BSN-Jobst (800) 537-1063
Website: www.jobst.com
Sells custom-made and ready-made vascular compression hosiery and lymphedema garments and offers a complete line of bandaging supplies.

Juzo (888) 255-1300
Website: www.juzousa.com
Manufactures compression therapy garments for lymphedema. Made with Lycra, Juzo garments are durable and latex-free. Juzo offers the widest variety of sizes and styles in compression arm sleeves, hand gloves/gauntlets, and stockings.

Medi-USA (800) 633-6334
Manufactures and sells a full line of ready-to-wear and custom-made compression sleeves and stockings, as well as therapeutic and support hosiery.

Sigvaris (800) 322-7744
Website: www.sigvaris.com
Manufactures and distributes medical compression socks, stockings, arm-sleeves, and bandages for veno-lymphatic disorders.

Specialized Garments

CircAid (800) 247-2243
Website: www.circaid.com
Offers garments to treat arm lymphedema, including both the Measure-Up 2001 Arm-Sleeve compression garment and the Silhouette, a soft foam sleeve that aids patients in self-bandaging. The products were designed by engineers, doctors, and therapists who understand lymphedema and its treatment.

Peninsula Medical, Inc., The Reid Sleeve People
(800) 29-EDEMA (800-293-3362)
Website: www.lymphedema.com or www.reidsleeve.com
Distributes specialty garments for the treatment and maintenance of lymphedema, including the Reid Sleeve, other soft-foam padded garments, the Contour Line, and OptiFlow Products.

MedAssist Group (800) 521-6664
Website: www.medassistgp.com
Distributes non-elastic limb-containment systems, including the ArmAssist Compression Sleeve. It also distributes the Anodyne Therapy System, a product providing infrared treatment.

Solaris, Inc (262) 821-6113
Website: www.swellingsolutions.com
Distributes Tribute garments, which are soft foam sleeves that aid in compression. It also distributes Swell Spots, smaller padding tools to apply to specific areas of the body.

Tri-D Corporation (866) 888-JOVI (866-888-5684)
Is the manufacturer and distributor of Jovi-Pak products, designed by lymphedema therapist Joanne Rovig. The company also offers self-care videos and other patient-education materials.

Other Equipment and Supplies

Flexitouch (866) 435-3948
Website: www.tactilesystems.com
The Flexitouch Lymphedema System is based on the physiological principles of manual lymph drainage. The Flexitouch Two Phase Preparation and Drainage process electronically inflates and deflates small chambers to prepare the trunk to receive and evacuate fluids, then concentrates therapy to drain the affected limb.

BioCompression Systems, Inc. (800) 888-0908
Website: www.biocompression.com
Distributor of the Seqeuential Circulator Lymphedema Pump, a gradient compression therapy lymphedema pump.

Global Medical Imports, Ltd. (800) 565-0868
E-mail: gmiltd_sampsonj@klis.com
A distributor of the compression pump known as the Lymphapress.

Lymphacare (800) 228-1801
Website: www.lymphacare.com
Distributes lymphedema products, including BioCompression Systems Sequential Circulator Lymphedema Pump, the Reid Sleeve, Med Assist specialty garments, and an infrared therapy system. Lymphacare will work with insurance companies to help with claims and reimbursement for lymphedema products.

Finding a Complementary-Care Provider
The websites of the following professional organizations feature directories of licensed practitioners in their resepective fields.

American Association of Naturopathic Physicians (AANP)
Website: www.naturopathic.org

National Certification Commission for Acupuncture and Oriental Medicine (NCCAOM)
Website: www.nccaom.org

index

CPSIA information can be obtained
at www.ICGtesting.com
Printed in the USA
JSHW051936221221
21473JS00001B/124